ILLUSTRATED
HUMAN EMBRYOLOGY

VOLUME III

NERVOUS SYSTEM
AND ENDOCRINE GLANDS

ILLUSTRATED HUMAN EMBRYOLOGY

VOLUME I: **EMBRYOGENESIS.**

VOLUME II: **ORGANOGENESIS.**

VOLUME III: **NERVOUS SYSTEM AND ENDOCRINE GLANDS.**

ILLUSTRATED HUMAN EMBRYOLOGY

VOLUME III

NERVOUS SYSTEM AND ENDOCRINE GLANDS

by

H. TUCHMANN-DUPLESSIS, M. D., Ph. D.
Professor, University of Paris Medical School,
Paris, France

M. AUROUX, M. D.
Assistant Professor, University of Paris Médical School,
Paris, France

P. HAEGEL, M. D.
Assistant Professor, University of Paris Medical School,
Paris, France

TRANSLATED BY

LUCILLE S. HURLEY, Ph. D.
Professor, University of California, Davis, California

SPRINGER-VERLAG
NEW YORK

CHAPMAN & HALL
LONDON

MASSON & C¹ᵉ, ÉDITEURS
PARIS

1975

ISBN : 0-387-90020-9

3-540-90020-9

0-412-12160-3

2-225-39622-1

INTRODUCTION

Embryology studies the succession of transformations undergone by the fertilized egg in the formation of a new individual. Development of the embryo is directed by morphogenetic mechanisms ruled by a strict chronology. Survival of the egg, its transport in the genital tract, and the adaptation of the maternal organism to its presence are controlled by hormonal actions.

Knowledge of these subjects is proving to be increasingly important for the medical practitioner. Such information helps to explain anatomic correlations; organ relationships also illuminate the etiology of numerous pathologic conditions. Disturbances of prenatal development engender congenital malformations and constitute an important cause of perinatal mortality and postnatal morbidity.

We are grateful to numerous students and colleagues whose cooperation has aided preparation of this book.

THE AUTHORS.

TRANSLATOR'S PREFACE

Translation of this work was undertaken in order to make available in English this excellent and unusual aid for the teaching and study of mammalian, primarily human, embryology.

This book emphasizes visual presentations. It combines the use of exceptionally clear and instructive drawings with photomicrographs and concise but complete text in an exposition of the dynamic aspects of development.

Thus, the three volumes of this book will be of help in preparation and review for students, research workers, medical practitioners such as obstetricians and pediatricians, and others who are concerned with embryology. Analysis of the precise timing of various stages of human development makes it especially useful for all who are interested in the study and prevention of congenital malformations.

The valuable assistance of Kenneth Thompson in the preparation of this work is gratefully acknowledged.

LUCILLE S. HURLEY.

FOREWORD TO VOLUME III

————————

Embryogenesis and general organogenesis have been dealt with in Volumes I and II. This third volume covers development of the nervous system, the sense organs, and the endocrine glands. The same general plan is followed as in the first two volumes, but there are also some special features because of the particular subject matter.

One of the characteristics of central nervous system development in man is that it summarizes the increasingly complex stages undergone by neural structures during the course of evolution. It therefore semed to us that embryological information should not be presented in isolation, that is, by discussing only ontogenesis. Instead, we have related such information to phylogenesis on the one hand, through simple notions of anatomy and comparative embryology, and on the other hand, to the anatomical and physiological states of the adult. Placed in this way between the elementary systems which precede them,· and the complex organization toward which they tend, the various stages of embryological development are integrated into a more easily understandable whole.

The sense organs and the endocrine glands form a functional system with the central nervous system as the pivot; with the sense organs, the nervous system insures rapid reactions to environmental stimuli; with the endocrine glands, it controls hormonal function and governs homeostasis; with both the sensory and endocrine systems, it regulates behavior. By showing the origin and morphogenesis of the pertinent structures, embryology provides better understanding of the relationships between these different functions.

Each chapter ends with a summary of the principal malformations found in man. Knowledge of normal and experimental embryology helps in understanding such pathology, which itself constitutes a special illustration of the major stages of development.

THE AUTHORS.

TABLE OF CONTENTS

SENSE ORGANS

ENDOCRINE GLANDS

NERVOUS SYSTEM

GENERAL ASPECTS

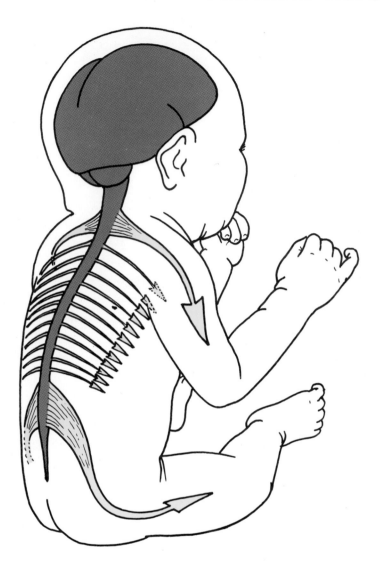

Fig. 1.

Diagrammatic view of nervous system of the infant. Violet : the central nervous system; yellow : peripheral nervous system; white : skin.

The nervous system as a whole, including spinal cord, brain, and peripheral nerves, is derived from the ectoderm. The primordial structure which gives rise to the nervous system, or neural ectoderm, appears very early, around the 17th day. It develops from the ectoderm in the dorsomedian region of the embryo, cephalic to Hensen's node and above the mesoderm. The latter, formed during gastrulation, induces formation of neural ectoderm from the overlying ectoderm.

During development, the neural ectoderm and the ectoderm separate: the ectoderm then forms the surface ectoderm, from which epidermis and certain sense organs originate.

ORIGIN OF NERVOUS SYSTEM

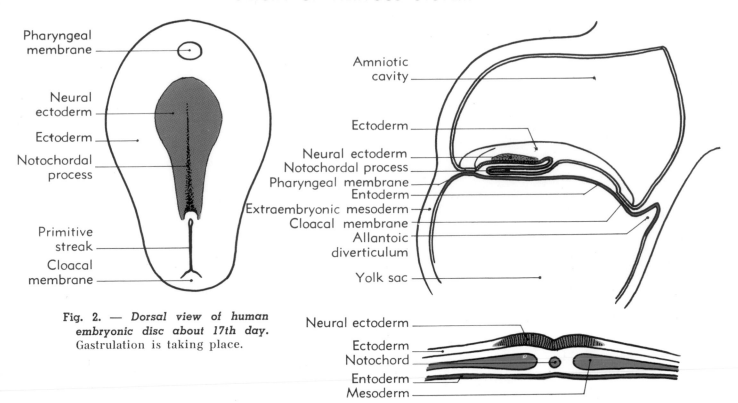

Pharyngeal membrane

Neural ectoderm

Ectoderm

Notochordal process

Primitive streak

Cloacal membrane

Fig. 2. — *Dorsal view of human embryonic disc about 17th day.* Gastrulation is taking place.

Amniotic cavity

Ectoderm
Neural ectoderm
Notochordal process
Pharyngeal membrane
Entoderm
Extraembryonic mesoderm
Cloacal membrane
Allantoic diverticulum

Yolk sac

Neural ectoderm
Ectoderm
Notochord
Entoderm
Mesoderm

Fig. 3. — *Sagittal section above, and cross section below, of an embryo at same stage of development.*

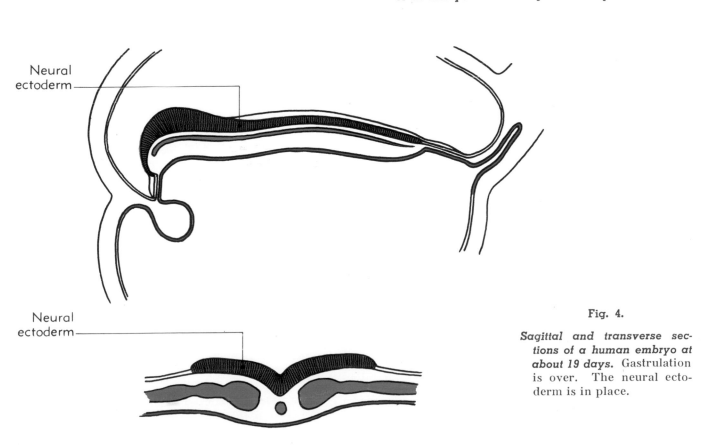

Neural ectoderm

Neural ectoderm

Fig. 4.

Sagittal and transverse sections of a human embryo at about 19 days. Gastrulation is over. The neural ectoderm is in place.

NEURULATION

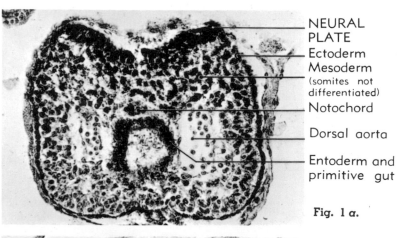

NEURAL
PLATE
Ectoderm
Mesoderm
(somites not
differentiated)
Notochord
Dorsal aorta
Entoderm and
primitive gut

Fig. 1 a.

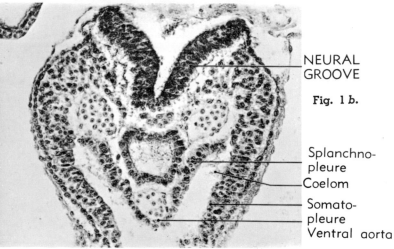

NEURAL
GROOVE

Fig. 1 b.

Splanchno-
pleure
Coelom
Somato-
pleure
Ventral aorta

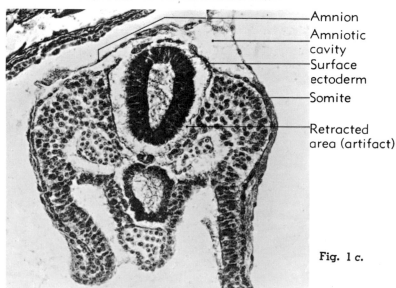

Amnion
Amniotic
cavity
Surface
ectoderm
Somite
Retracted
area (artifact)

Fig. 1 c.

Neurulation is the transformation of the ectoderm overlying the notochord into the neural tube flanked by two longitudinal formations, the neural crests.

Formation of the neural tube

Formation of the neural tube consists of three successive stages:

— **The neural plate** results from differentiation and thickening of the ectoderm overlying the notochord. It is wider at the cephalic end than at the caudal end. In man, it is formed about the 17th day, that is, before the appearance of the first somites.

At the periphery, the ectoderm remains thin (fig. 1 *a*).

— **The neural groove** results from invagination of the plate (fig. 1 *b*).

— **The neural tube** results from fusion of the edges of the groove. This stage is also called the neurula stage. The ectoderm is then separate from the nervous tissue: this is the surface ectoderm. Between the two, mesenchymal cells gradually infiltrate.

The three stages, plate, groove, and tube, coexist at the same time in different regions of the embryo. In fact, closure of the neural groove, which begins about the 21st day in man, is accomplished first in the middle part of the embryo, and then progresses toward the two ends (fig. 2 and 3). This middle region, although equidistant from the cephalic and caudal extremities, represents the future brain region.

For a relatively short time, two orifices persist at each end of the tube, the anterior and posterior neuropores. The anterior achieves its definitive form about the 26th day, the posterior about the 28th day (fig. 2).

Fig. 1 *a, b, c.* — *The three stages of neurulation in the rat.* 11-day embryo (× 170).

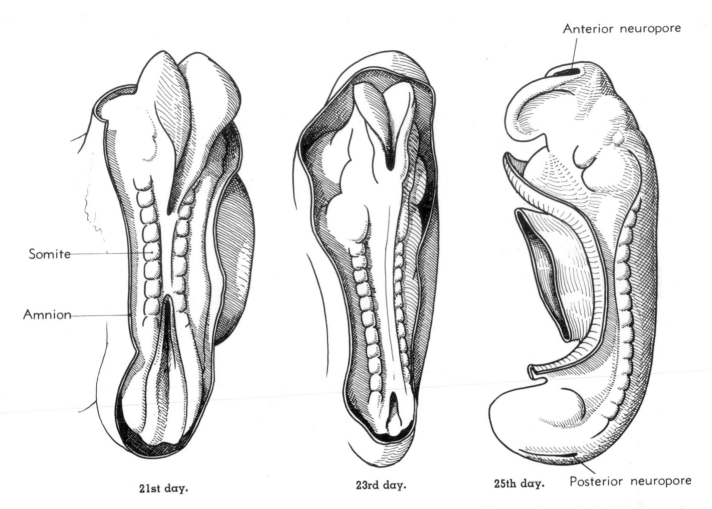

Anterior neuropore

Somite

Amnion

21st day.   23rd day.   25th day.   Posterior neuropore

Fig. 2. — *Closure of neural tube in human embryo.*

The cephalic end of the neural tube is larger than its caudal end; the outlines of the cerebral vesicles are visible even before complete closure of the cephalic groove has occurred (fig. 2).

In higher vertebrates and man, the terminal caudal portion of the neural tube originates in a different manner from the cephalic part. The neural primordium of the caudal flexure is initially a solid cord, and only secondarily hollows out to form an ependymal cavity. Later, this regresses.

Neurulation contributes to the cephalocaudal flexion * of the embryo. The extensive proliferation of nervous tissue causes curvature of the embryo on its longitudinal axis (fig. 3). A progressive dorsal flexion results in raising and isolating the embryo from its membranes (see Vol. I).

* TRANSLATOR'S NOTE: Franch embryologists use the term "délimitation" to denote the overall process involving formation of the body cylinder and cephalocaudal flexion, and leading from the flat embryonic disc to assumption of the basic embryonic body form. The terms cephalocaudal flexion, or flexion, will be used here.

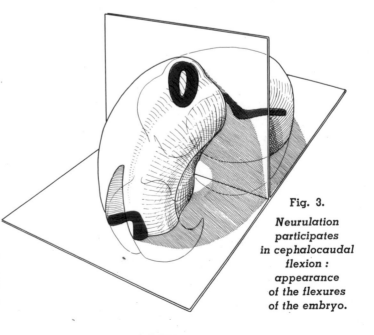

Fig. 3.

Neurulation participates in cephalocaudal flexion : appearance of the flexures of the embryo.

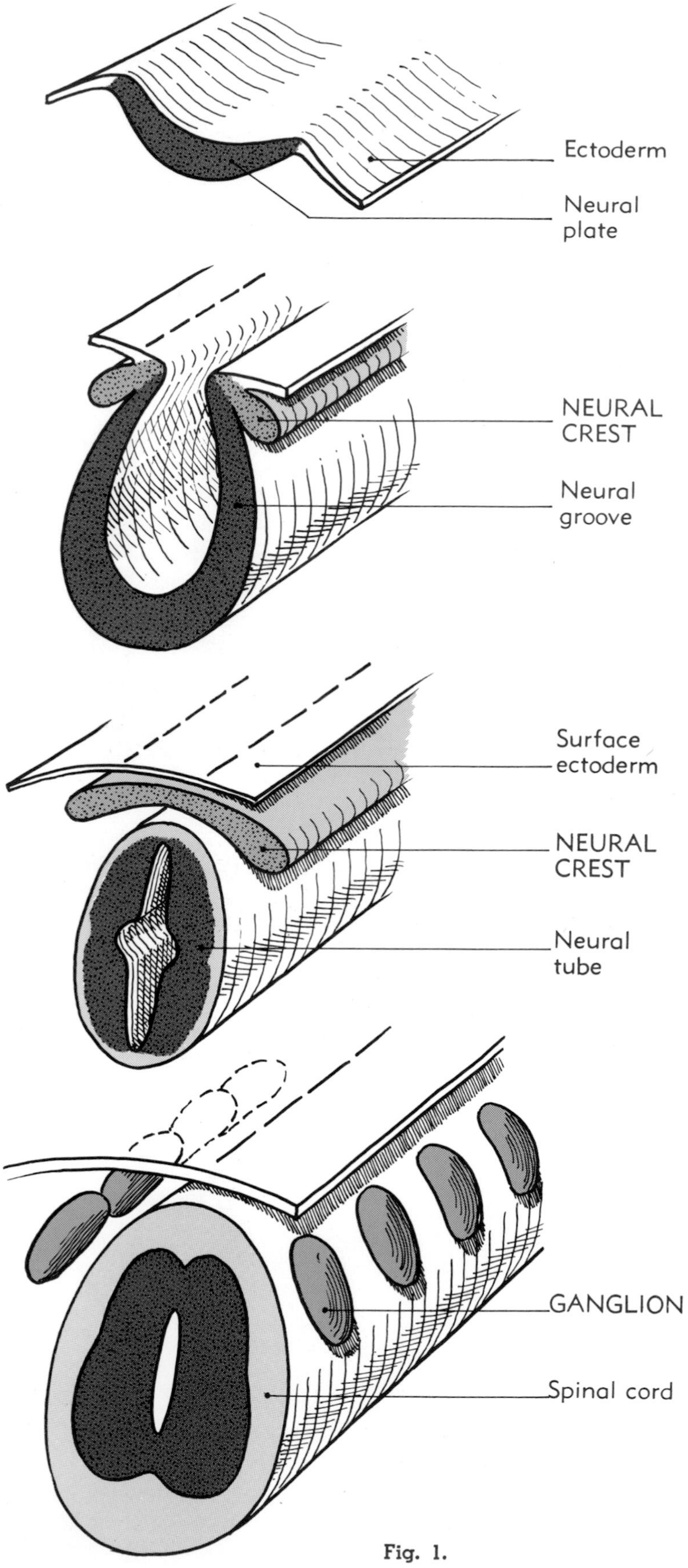

Ectoderm

Neural plate

NEURAL CREST

Neural groove

Surface ectoderm

NEURAL CREST

Neural tube

GANGLION

Spinal cord

Fig. 1.

II. — THE NEURAL CRESTS

Before complete closure of the neural groove, some cells become detached from the region where the neural tube borders on the ectoderm. These groups of cells are the neural crests.

After closure, the crests are distinct from both the neural tube and the ectoderm. They then form longitudinal tracts which extend from the caudal end to the midbrain regions of the neural tube.

The neural crests soon fragment and give rise to primordia of the ganglia. This segmentation corresponds to that of the somites: each ganglionic primordium corresponds to a muscle primordium. The ganglia later give rise to general sensory innervation, and the corresponding level of the spinal cord furnishes motor innervation of the muscles (fig. 3 and 4, p. 23).

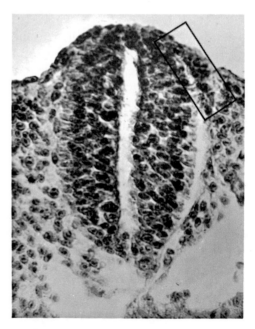

Fig. 2. — *Neural crest of an 11-day rat embryo;* easily visible at right (box), less clear at left (× 300).

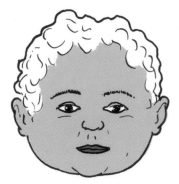

Fig. 3.

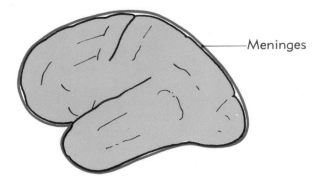

Fig. 4.

DERIVATIVES OF NEURAL CRESTS

— Ectomesenchyme (1) :
  - — dermis of head (fig. 3);
  - — soft meninges (fig. 4);
  - — skleton and perhaps musculature of branchial arches.
— Cells of spinal ganglia, ganglia of sympathetic and parasympathetic systems, including the adrenal medulla (fig. 5).
— Schwann cells forming the myelin sheaths of peripheral nerves.
— Pigment cells, particularly of the skin (fig. 7).

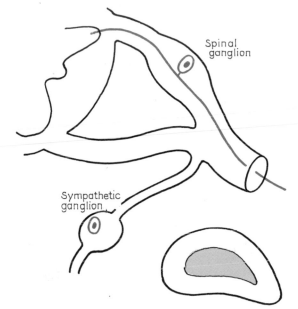

Fig. 5.

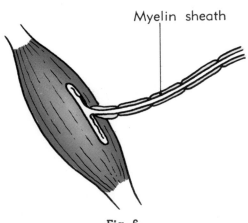

Fig. 6.

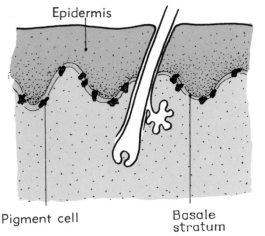

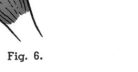

Fig. 7.

(1) The ectomesenchyme results from mesenchymal differentiation of neuroblastic cells; it is therefore of ectodermal origin.

INDUCTION OF THE

The various phases of neurulation are induced by the notochord and the parachordal mesoderm (inductors) from the overlying ectoderm (competent). Induction also plays a part in the subsequent development of the nervous system.

Activity of inductors is not uniform: there is a cephalocaudal gradient. The trunk areas of the notochord and parachordal mesoderm induce formation of spinal cord, while their anterior extremities induce the posterior and middle parts of the brain (rhombencephalon and mesencephalon). The prosencephalon is induced by a specific structure situated in front of the notochord, the prechordal plate. This term designates a mixed mesoentodermal structure, resulting from fusion of the extreme anterior end of the notochordal process with the adjacent entodermal layers (1). The competent tissue is then represented by the anterior end of the neural tube.

During its development, the neural tube in turn induces formation of the posterior arch of the vertebrae and of the cranial vault. It also enters into development of the face, the eye, and the nose.

Many abnormalities can occur in such a complex mechanism since either induction or competence can be defective at each step.

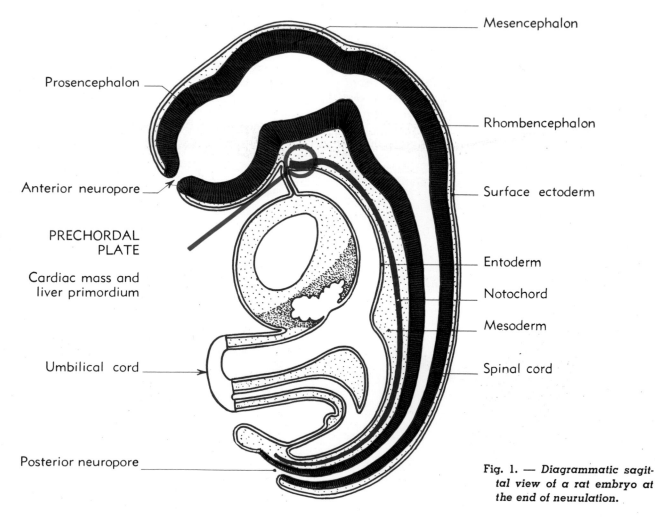

Fig. 1. — *Diagrammatic sagittal view of a rat embryo at the end of neurulation.*

(1) See figure 5, page 13, role of the entoderm in hemichords.

NERVOUS SYSTEM

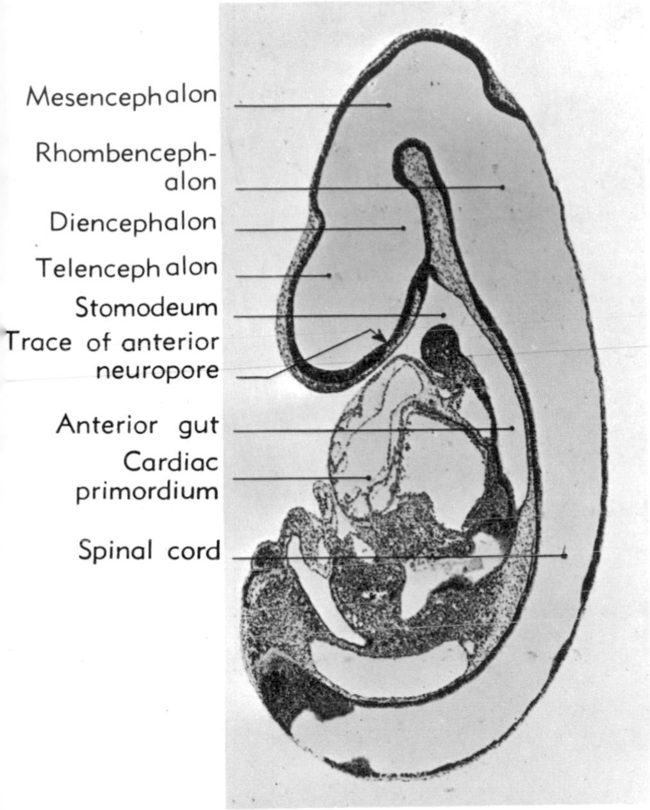

Mesencephalon

Rhombenceph-
alon

Diencephalon

Telencephalon

Stomodeum

Trace of anterior
neuropore

Anterior gut

Cardiac
primordium

Spinal cord

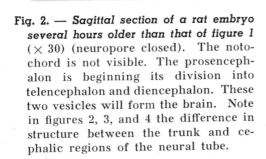

Fig. 2. — *Sagittal section of a rat embryo several hours older than that of figure 1* (× 30) (neuropore closed). The notochord is not visible. The prosencephalon is beginning its division into telencephalon and diencephalon. These two vesicles will form the brain. Note in figures 2, 3, and 4 the difference in structure between the trunk and cephalic regions of the neural tube.

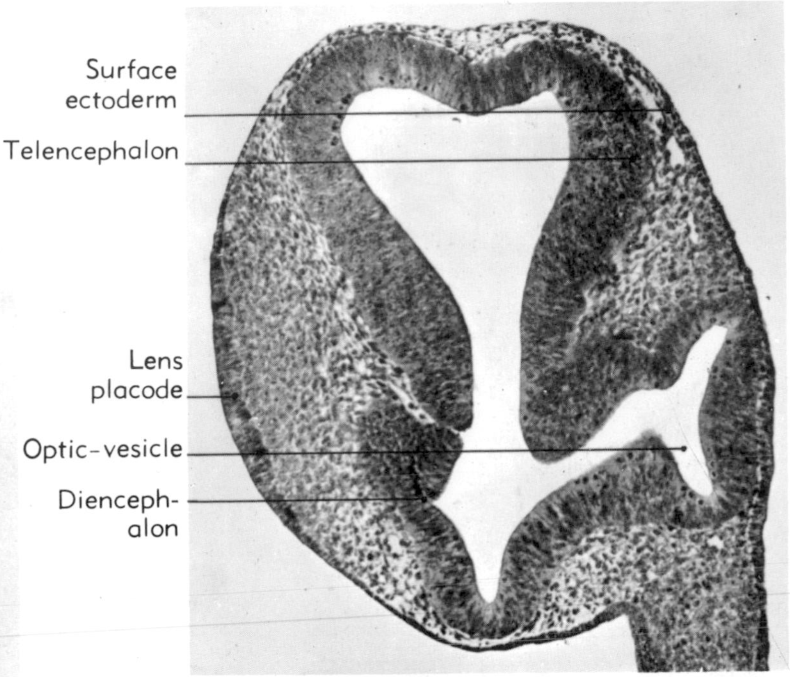

Surface
ectoderm

Telencephalon

Lens
placode

Optic-vesicle

Dienceph-
alon

Fig. 3. — *Cross section of prosencephalon.* Only one of the two optic primordia is seen, because the section is not perfectly frontal (× 110).

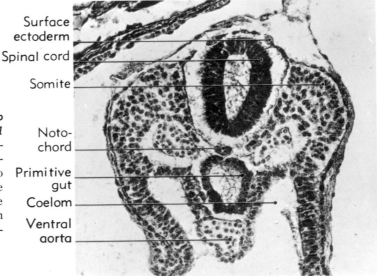

Surface
ectoderm

Spinal cord

Somite

Noto-
chord

Primitive
gut

Coelom

Ventral
aorta

Fig. 4. — *Cross section of spinal cord* (× 170).

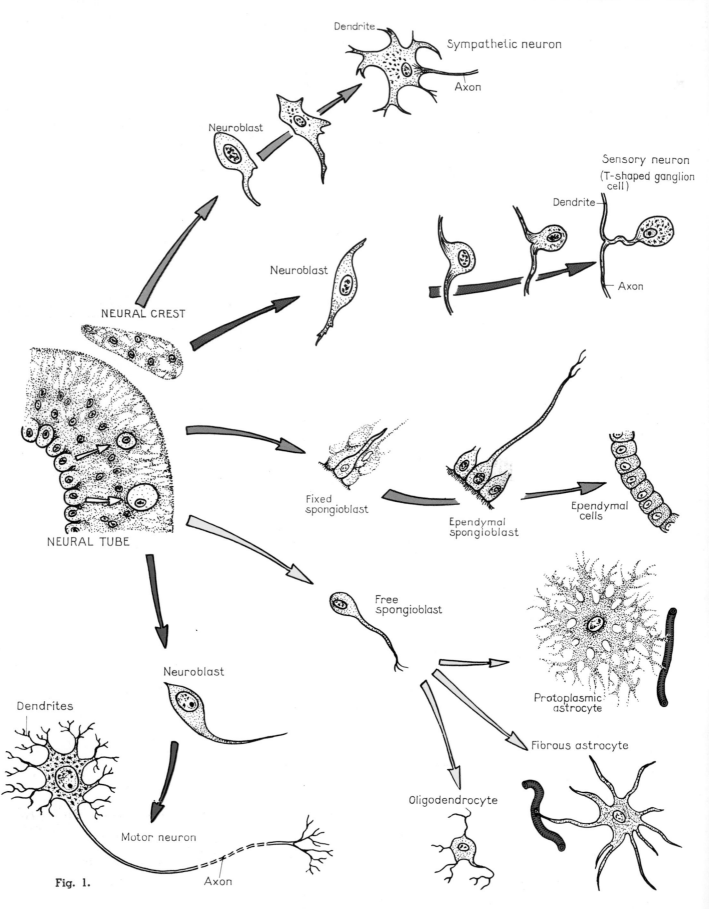

Fig. 1.

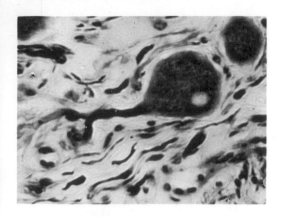

Fig. 2. — *T-shaped cell of spinal ganglion* ($\times$ 425).

Histogenesis is the combination of the processes of multiplication and differentiation which are undergone by the cells of the 3 embryonic layers. It results in specialized cells organzed to form the tissues of the adult organism. It is especially complex in regard to nervous tissue.

Histogenesis begins with closure of the neural tube. It involves:

a) **The neural tube.** The epithelial cells bordering the lumen of the tube form the germinal region which produces two categories of cells (fig. 1):

— large-sized cells which migrate progressively towards the periphery: these are the *neuroblasts*, future neurons;

— smaller cells, the *spongioblasts*, which follow two different paths: some are fixed and give rise to the ependymal cells; the others are free, migrate toward the periphery and give rise to the neuroglial cells (1).

Some cells have both neuronal and neuroglial potentialities, and could differentiate in either direction.

b) **The neural crest** (fig. 1). This furnishes two kinds of neuroblasts:

— bipolar cells which develop without migrating (future spinal ganglion cells);

— multipolar cells which migrate interiorly (future sympathetic ganglia cells).

Transformation of the cells into neurons includes:

— enlargement of nuclear volume;

— appearance of Nissl bodies (cytoplasmic RNA);

— formation of processes: first axons, then dendrites (fig. 1, 2, and 3).

Histogenesis of nervous tissue continues for a long time, especially in the higher nervous structures. Thus, in man, most of the neurons of the cerebral cortex are present at birth, but the definitive establishment of interneuronal connections extends over several years.

Myelination follows histogenesis. It occurs later and persists longer as the systems are phylogenetically more recent:

— for peripheral nerves, myelination is accomplished by Schwann cells; it begins in the 4th month of fetal life;

— for the fibers in the interior of the CNS, it is the neuroglial cells (oligodendrites) derived from the neural tube which furnish the myelin sheath. Central myelination begins about the same time as that of peripheral nerves, about the 4th month of fetal life. It appears in the 6th month in the vestibulospinal tract and in the 7th month in the rubrospinal tract. Some motor fibers coming from upper cerebral centers, the pyramidal tract for example, are myelinated during the first two years after birth. The slowness of this process and the correlations between myelination and final establishment of functional ability partly explain the long duration of psychomotor development in the child.

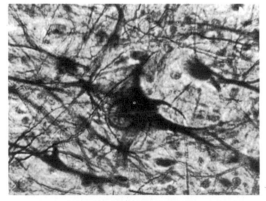

Fig. 3. — *Motor neuron of anterior horn of the spinal cord* ($\times$ 425).

(1) Microglial cells are classified as neuroglia. Actually, these cells are not of neural but of mesenchymal origin. They are macrophagic cells of the histiocyte system, with neural localization, brought into the CNS by blood vessels. There is some evidence, however, that the microglia could be ectomesenchymal.

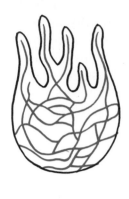

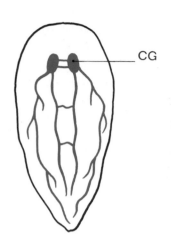

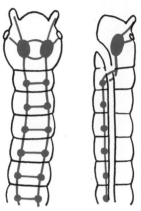

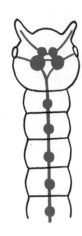

Fig. 1. — *Coelenterates (Sea anemones).* Diffuse neural network.

Fig. 2. — *Primitive worms* (Convoluta). The nervous system is more concentrated and shows the beginning of cephalization (cerebral ganglia CG). It is approaching a central nervous system (CNS) organization. However, it is ventral and without a cavity.

Fig. 3. — *Lower annelids* (Serpula). Concentration increased. Appearance of segmentation (metamerization). Ventral CNS without cavity.

Fig. 4. — *Superior annelids* (Nereis). Transverse concentration. The cerebral ganglia are specialized (1, olfaction; 2, vision). CNS still ventral and without cavity.

Vertebrates are distinguished from other groups of animals by several characteristics, principally concerning the spinal cord and nervous system:

1. Presence of a dorsal notochord surrounded by mesodermal tissue which gives rise to the vertebral column in adults of most species.

2. A tubular nervous system, dorsal to the cord, concentrated in the midline and considerably developed cephalically (cephalization).

Specific aspects of these differences may be demonstrated through *comparative anatomy:*

— progressive concentration of the nervous system and beginning of cephalization (fig. 1 to 4);
— appearance and changes in segmentation (fig. 3 and 4);
— appearance of notochord and nervous system of vertebrates (fig. 5, 6, and 7).

Comparative embryology illuminates various phases of this evolution. In all animals which have one, the nervous system derives from the ectoderm (1). However, the extent and pathways of its development differ between the invertebrates and the vertebrates.

1. **In invertebrates,** that is, before the evolutionary appearance of the cord, neural organization seems to depend on sensory surface ectoderm cells.

— In **coelenterates,** these cells are diffuse and the nervous system itself is diffuse.
— In **worms,** the sensory cells concentrate in certain regions of the individual and the nervous system follows a parallel development: it becomes a central nervous system. At the anterior end of the animal, sensory concentration is especially clear. Nervous concentration is also greater at this location than elsewhere (fig. 2 to 4). Thus, strict parallelism is observed between anterior concentration of sensory and nervous cells. Progressive localization of sensory cells seems, in the same way, to be responsible for the segmental nervous concentrations forming the metameric ganglia (fig. 3 and 4).

(1) Some ganglion cells, principally intestinal, are of entodermal origin.

NERVOUS SYSTEM

2. *In vertebrates,* the mesoderm determines development of both the nervous system and the sense organs. The nervous system is thus relatively independent of the sensory organization. Certain sense organs are even derived directly from it, such as the eye and the general sensory receptors.

Fig. 5. — *Hemichordates* (Enteropneusts). Dorsal tubular CNS. Solid ventral CNS. No cord in the strict sense, but a cephalodorsal diverticulum of the intestine which corresponds to a dorsal nervous tube. This is incompletely separated from the overlying ectoderm from which it is derived.

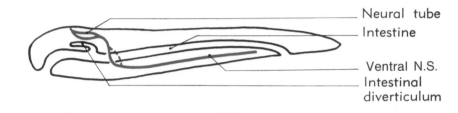

Neural tube
Intestine

Ventral N.S.
Intestinal diverticulum

Fig. 6. — *Prochordates* (Amphioxus). Dorsal cord. Dorsal tubular CNS, entirely developed from dorsal ectoderm. The anterior vesicle represents a true rudimentary brain. A ventral CNS no longer exists.

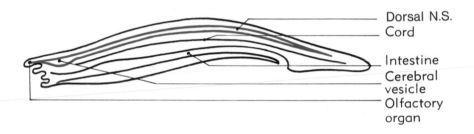

Dorsal N.S.
Cord

Intestine
Cerebral vesicle
Olfactory organ

Fig. 7. — *Vertebrates.* In the less evolved vertebrates, such as fishes, the 5 neural vesicles presage the great cephalization of the higher vertebrates (fig. 1, p. 60). During this slow progression, the role of the prechordal plate is essential. It induces the brain as such; man offers the most developed example.

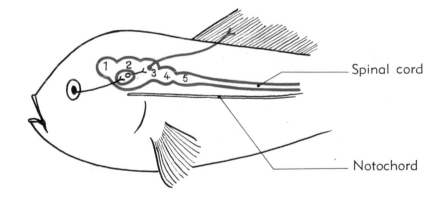

Spinal cord

Notochord

Thus, during the course of evolution, relationships between the nervous system and the sense organs are modified. In invertebrates, the nervous system seems to be only an accessory to the sensory system. In vertebrates, on the contrary, its importance becomes so great that everything seems to be organized around it and for it. These characteristics find their most complete expression in man.

Appearance of the mesoderm, which seems to group together inductive capabilities, marks an important stage in the genesis of these transformations.

SPINAL CORD

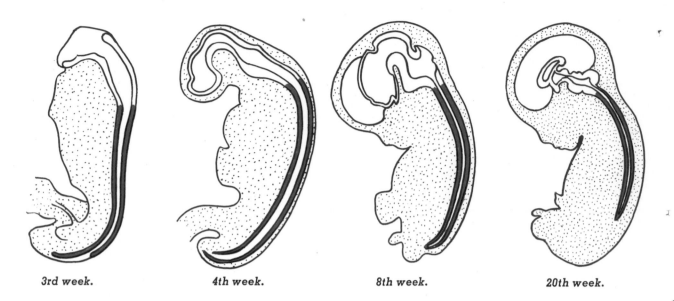

3rd week.   4th week.   8th week.   20th week.

The spinal cord occupies the dorsal and median part of the embryo. It is directly caudal to the medulla, the most caudal portion of the brain (fig. 1 and 2).

It is surrounded by the meninges and lodged in the bony vertebral canal. Its axial cavity is the ependymal canal.

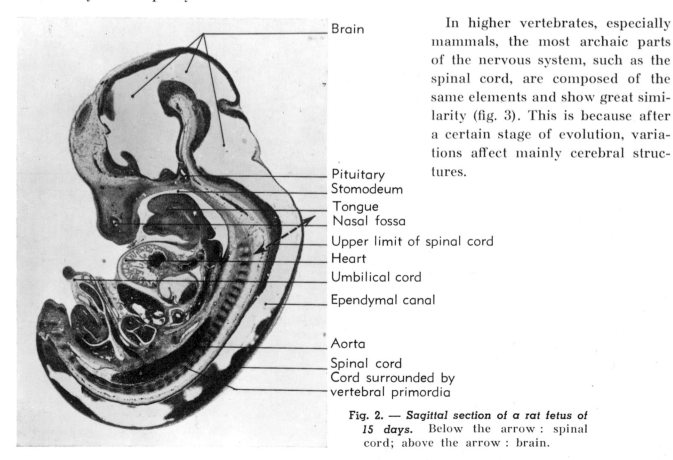

Brain

Pituitary
Stomodeum
Tongue
Nasal fossa
Upper limit of spinal cord
Heart
Umbilical cord
Ependymal canal

Aorta
Spinal cord
Cord surrounded by
vertebral primordia

In higher vertebrates, especially mammals, the most archaic parts of the nervous system, such as the spinal cord, are composed of the same elements and show great similarity (fig. 3). This is because after a certain stage of evolution, variations affect mainly cerebral structures.

Fig. 2. — *Sagittal section of a rat fetus of 15 days.* Below the arrow : spinal cord; above the arrow : brain.

GENERAL CHARACTERISTICS

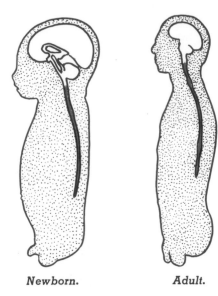

Newborn.   *Adult.*

Fig. 1. — *Relative size of central nervous system and of the body at different stages of development.*

The size of the spinal cord varies with the age of the fetus. Its relative volume, large to begin with, diminishes progressively in relation to the total volume of the central nervous system (fig. 1), and especially in relation to the total body size.

Surface ectoderm

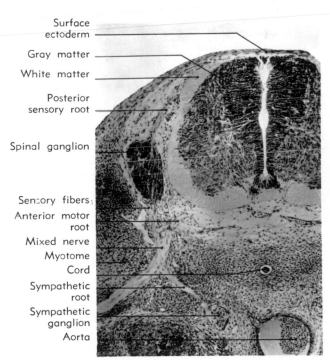

Surface ectoderm
Gray matter
White matter
Posterior sensory root
Spinal ganglion
Sensory fibers
Anterior motor root
Mixed nerve
Myotome
Cord
Sympathetic root
Sympathetic ganglion
Aorta

Fig. 3 a. — *Cross section of rat fetus of 15 days. Dorsal level (× 90).*

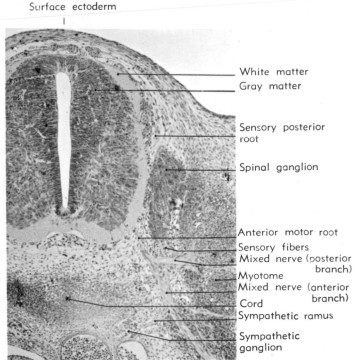

White matter
Gray matter
Sensory posterior root
Spinal ganglion
Anterior motor root
Sensory fibers
Mixed nerve (posterior branch)
Myotome
Mixed nerve (anterior branch)
Cord
Sympathetic ramus
Sympathetic ganglion

Fig. 3 b. — *Cross section of human fetus about 45 days. Dorsal level (× 65).*

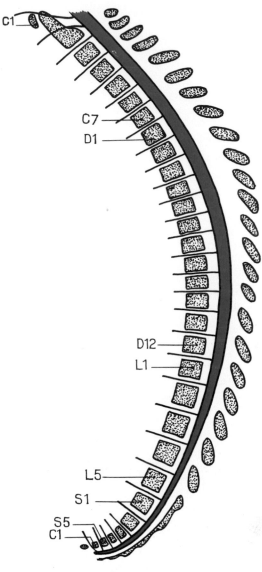

Fig. 1. — *Spinal cord of fetus before 4th month.*

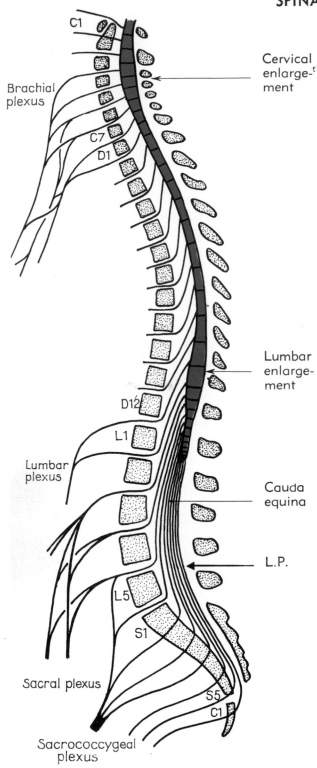

Fig. 2. — *Spinal cord of adult*
(according to J. DELMAS and A. DELMAS).

In the beginning, the neural tube and the vertebral canal develop in an almost parallel way. The spinal cord occupies the entire length of the canal and perpendicular to it, the spinal nerves emerge between the vertebral bodies (fig. 1).

In the 4th month, growth of the neural tube slows down considerably, while that of the vertebral canal continues.

CORD

Because of this:

— the spinal cord no longer occupies the entire length of the vertebral canal;

— the roots of the lumbar and sacral nerves, originally horizontal, are dragged down by the vertebral canal. They become long and vertical, and form the cauda equina (horse's tail) below the spinal cord (2nd lumbar vertebra in the adult, fig. 2).

The spinal cord is attached to the end of the spine by only a thin strand, the *filum terminale,* which is the atrophied caudal portion of the neural tube.

Below the second lumbar vertebra, generally between L4 and L5, a lumbar puncture may be made without danger. At this level, there is no spinal cord, only meninges, cerebro-spinal fluid, and the mobile nerves of the cauda equina through which the needle will slide (fig. 2, L.P.).

At two points the spinal cord widens to form the cervical and lumbar enlargements, which are located at the level of origin of nerves of the branchial plexus to the arm and the lumbosacral plexus to the leg. The enlargements contain numerous neuroblasts, in accordance with the rich innervation of the upper and lower limbs.

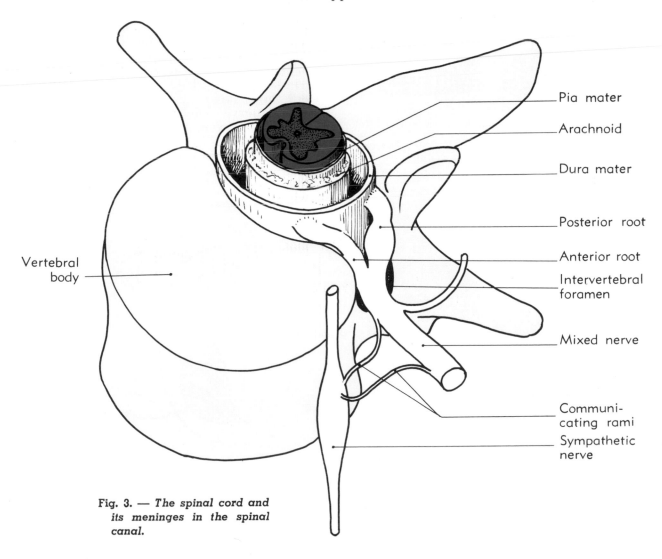

Pia mater

Arachnoid

Dura mater

Posterior root

Anterior root

Intervertebral foramen

Mixed nerve

Communi-cating rami

Sympathetic nerve

Vertebral body

Fig. 3. — *The spinal cord and its meninges in the spinal canal.*

When the neural tube is formed, the cells of the germinating epithelium proliferate actively. They form the thick, multilayered, periependymal wall of the neural tube (fig. 1). Then the cells migrate toward the periphery. They group into clusters forming the **mantle layer,** primordium of the gray matter. Simultaneously, they differentiate. The ventral clusters form the **basal plate,** primordium of the anterior, motor, horn. The dorsal clusters form the **alar plate,** primordium of the sensory posterior horn. The basal and alar plates are separated by a groove, the *sulcus limitans.* Opposite this, the sympathetic cells of the horn develop laterally, sensory cells dorsally, and motor cells ventrally (fig. 2 and 2*a*).

The mantle layer is surrounded by the **marginal layer.** The latter, very poor in cells, is composed mainly of myelinated nerve fibers; it is the future white matter (see p. 25).

Development and differentiation of these cell clusters bring about enlargements and peripheral grooves, while at the center, the cavity diminishes and its cells form the ependyma. Mitotic activity of the ependymal epithelium decreases progressively (fig. 4 and 5).

The axons of the cells of the anterior horn and of the ventral portion of the lateral horn form the anterior motor root of the spinal nerve. The cells of the spinal ganglia each have a peripheral prolongation, the dendrite, and a central prolongation, the axon (fig. 2 and 2*a*). These two prolongations, contiguous at first, give a T-shaped appearance to the ganglion cell (see p. 11). The dendrite grows toward the periphery and forms the sensory portion of the mixed nerve. The axon grows toward the posterior portion of the tube and forms the sensory (fig. 2 to 5). The fibers of this root terminate in the posterior somatic or sympathetic gray matter (fig. 2*a*), or reach the brain, going through the white matter. The white matter thickens as the

Ectoderm

Germinating
epithelium

Neural crest

Periependymal
zone

Myotome

Sclerotome

Notochord

Dorsal aorta

Posterior
cardinal vein

Mesonephric
vesicle

Root of
mesentery

Hindgut

Fig. 1. — *Human embryo about 25 days,* dorsal level (× 75). The neural groove is about to close. The medullary canal is wide and the wall relatively narrow. There is still no apparent cellular differentiation.

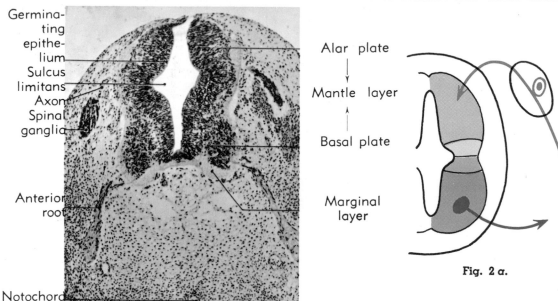

Germinating
epithelium

Sulcus
limitans

Axon

Spinal
ganglia

Anterior
root

Notochord

Alar plate
↓
Mantle layer
↑
Basal plate

Marginal
layer

Fig. 2 a.

Fig. 2. — *Human embryo about 35 days,* dorsal level (× 70). The motor roots develop a little before the sensory roots.

SPINAL CORD

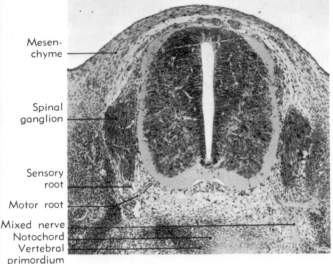

Mesen-
chyme

Spinal
ganglion

Sensory
root

Motor root

Mixed nerve
Notochord
Vertebral
primordium

Fig. 3. — Human embryo about 45 days,
dorsal level (× 50). Motor and sensory
roots constitute the mixed nerve.

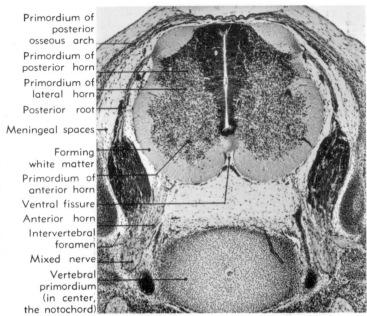

Primordium of
posterior
osseous arch

Primordium of
posterior horn

Primordium of
lateral horn

Posterior root

Meningeal spaces

Forming
white matter

Primordium of
anterior horn

Ventral fissure

Anterior horn

Intervertebral
foramen

Mixed nerve

Vertebral
primordium
(in center,
the notochord)

Fig. 4. — Human embryo, about 60 days, dorsal level (× 45).
The spinal cord is getting its shape. The fissures appear.

number of sensory (ascending) and motor (descending) fibers increases.

Fibers crossing over from both sides of the cord form the commissures which connect the right and left parts of the gray matter (fig. 5).

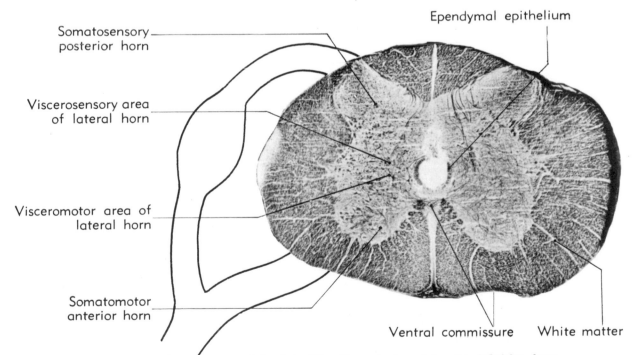

Somatosensory
posterior horn

Ependymal epithelium

Viscerosensory area
of lateral horn

Visceromotor area of
lateral horn

Somatomotor
anterior horn

Ventral commissure   White matter

Fig. 5. — Newborn cat, dorsal level (× 35). The spinal cord has its definitive form.
The gray matter with its anterior and posterior horns rich in cells can be recognized,
as well as the white matter containing only fibers. (In this silver nitrate stained
preparation, the white matter appears dark.) The ependymal canal has become
very small in relation to the total size of the spinal cord, and the former germinating
zone constitutes the ependymal epithelium.

The autonomic nervous system (ANS) is concerned with those processes normally beyond voluntary control and for the most part beneath consciousness. It differs in this way from the voluntary central nervous system; however, it is under the control of centers in the CNS and cannot function as an independent unit.

It is composed of two portions, anatomically and physiologically distinct: the **sympathetic** and **parasympathetic** systems. These systems are **essentially motor systems,** since the sensory afferent nerves (with a few exceptions) follow the ordinary sensory pathways (fig. 2).

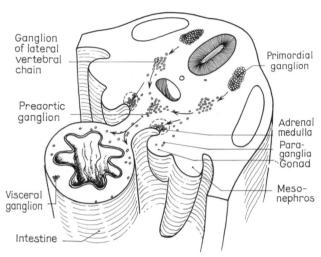

Fig. 1 (according to GIROUD and LELIÈVRE).

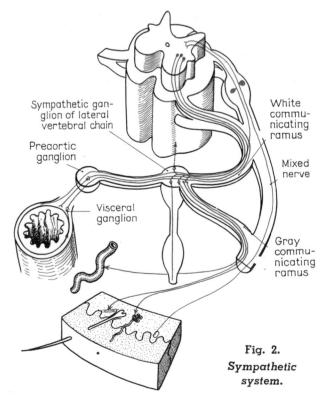

Fig. 2.
Sympathetic system.

In red : motor pathways; in blue : sensory pathways.

I. — THE SYMPATHETIC SYSTEM

About the 5th week of development, cells from the neural crest and the ventral portion of the neural tube migrate from each side of the spinal cord. These are the future sympathetic cells, or sympathetic neuroblasts (fig. 1 and 2, p. 130). Some detach themselves from the tube and arrange themselves along the motor root.

In this way they form two chains of sympathetic ganglia (fig. 1 and 2, and fig. 3, p. 15). These ganglia are segmental or metameric, but, in contrast to the spinal ganglia, they are connected to each other by the axons of some cells. The resulting interconnected ganglionated cord forms the lateral vertebral sympathetic chain which extends from the cervical to the lumbosacral region.

Some of the sympathetic neuroblasts migrate even farther ventrally to form preaortic ganglia such as the solar (celiac) plexus and visceral ganglia such as the myenteric plexus of Auerbach and the submucous plexus of Meissner (fig. 1 and 2). The ultimate nerve network in which this system terminates in the intestinal wall has the same origin.

While the ganglia are forming, fibers coming from the visceral motor zone of the medulla make synapses with the sympathetic neuroblasts of one of the three ganglionic levels; these are the preganglionic fibers. These fibers are myelinated; their path, from the spinal nerves to the sympathetic ganglia, constitutes the *white communicating rami.*

The axons of sympathetic neuroblasts constitute the unmyelinated postganglionic fibers (fig. 2). These fibers leave the ganglion system at one of its three levels. The fibers innervat-

NERVOUS SYSTEM

ing diffuse structures such as peripheral vessels, hair follicles, and sweat glands arise from ganglia of the lateral chain and reach the spinal nerve by the gray communicating ramus. The fibers innervating the eye, the heart, the lungs and the digestive tract originate in the three ganglion levels.

II. — THE PARASYMPATHETIC SYSTEM

The parasympathetic system is less extensive than the sympathetic. Preganglionic fibers arise only in certain centers of the sacral spinal cord and of the cerebral trunk. They follow the path of the corresponding nerves (fig. 3). Like the sympathetic neuroblasts, ganglion cells come from the neural crest and neural tube, but only at the level of the preganglionic fibers. Their long migration takes them to the viscera; all the parasympathetic ganglia are preaortic or visceral.

Some parasympathetic receptors: carotid and aortic bodies. — The carotid and aortic bodies are mesenchymal chemoreceptors, innervated by the glosso-pharyngeal (IX) nerve. The neurosensory cells which make up these structures are of parasympathetic origin: they migrate along the ninth nerve from the neural crest or tube.

III. — PHYSIOLOGICAL SIGNIFICANCE OF ANS

The postganglionic neuron of the sympathetic system is adrenergic, while that of the parasympathetic system is cholinergic. Antagonism of these two systems contributes to the maintenance of equilibrium of involuntary functions. The entire system is under the control of the hypothalamus which coordinates information relating to the involuntary functions.

IV. — PATHOLOGY

Abnormal organogenesis of the ANS is responsible for certain problems especially involving the digestive tract, such as Hirschsprung's disease (megacolon or congenital dilatation of the colon, with anomalies of Meissner's and Auerbach's plexes).

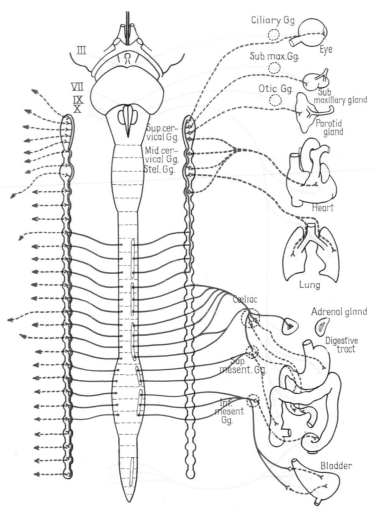

Fig. 3. — *The sympathetic (in red) and the parasympathetic (in yellow) systems.* All organs have a double innervation. Straight lines : preganglionic fibers; dotted lines : postganglionic fibers. At left, somatic distribution of sympathetic system (according to STRONG and ELWYN).

Metameric organization appears for the first time in the annelids (fig. 3, p. 12). Each metamere carries a pair of nerve ganglia, a cutaneous component, a group of muscles, and various other mesodermal derivatives: visceral, vascular, etc. The cutaneous portion sends sensory afferents to the ganglia, which respond by stimulating motor efferents to the muscles. There is thus an anatomical and physiological unit which theoretically could function autonomously.

This unit is more advanced in organization than the diffuse structures of the primitive invertebrates (fig. 1 and 2, p. 12).

Ascending the scale of invertebrates, towards insects, for example, neighboring ganglionic pairs tend to fuse. The coresponding metameres interweave and coordinate their functions. The independence of each segment is sacrificed for the welfare of the whole.

In vertebrates and man, the neural tube-neural crest combination replaces the essentially ganglionic system of the invertebrates. However, metamerization remains, especially in the trunk (fig. 1).

Metamerization manifests itself first by aggregation of the paraxial mesoderm into somites. The first somites appear in the posterior portion of the cephalic region and segmentation progresses toward the caudal region.

In a parallel way, the neural crests break up, producing the ganglionic primordia which correspond, one to one, to the lateral somites (fig. 3). The cutaneous areas opposite the somites constitute the dermatomes. The spinal cord itself does not divide. Nevertheless, it can be considered virtually segmented, for a medullary level or neuromere corresponds functionally to each ganglion and somite level (fig. 4). These various elements: dermatomes, ganglia, neuromere, and myotomes (derived from somites) form a metamere.

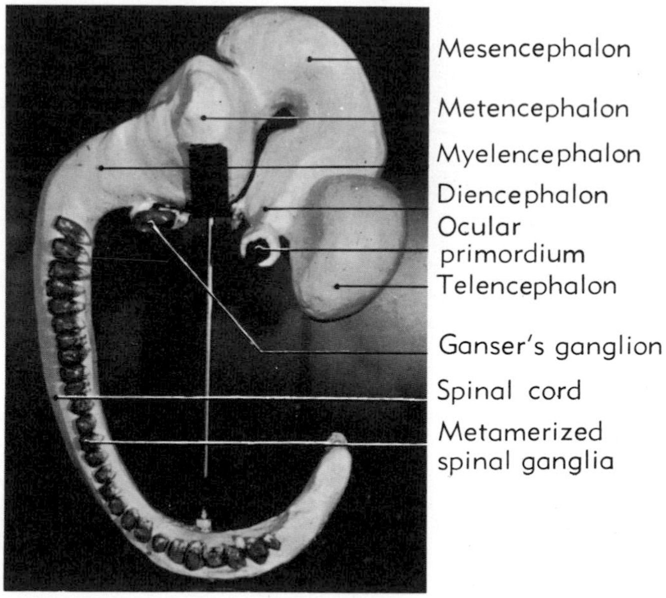

Mesencephalon
Metencephalon
Myelencephalon
Diencephalon
Ocular primordium
Telencephalon
Ganser's ganglion
Spinal cord
Metamerized spinal ganglia

Fig. 1. — *Reconstruction of CNS of a 14-day rat embryo.*

ORGANIZATION

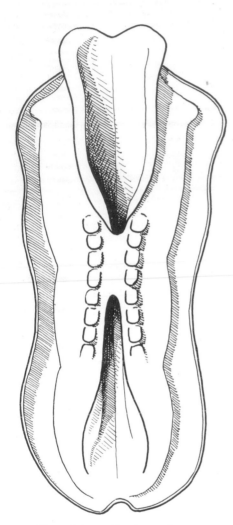

Fig. 2. — *Somites, demonstrating metamerization.* Human embryo, 7-somite stage (about 22 days).

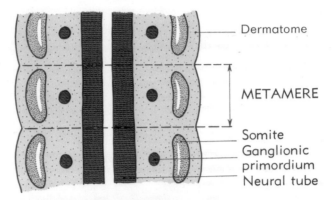

Dermatome

METAMERE

Somite
Ganglionic primordium
Neural tube

Fig. 3. — *The anatomic metamere.* Parallel section of dorsal plane of embryo (according to GIROUD).

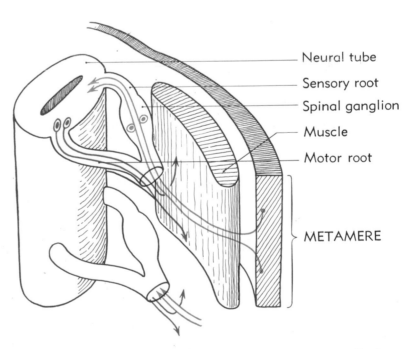

Neural tube
Sensory root
Spinal ganglion
Muscle
Motor root

METAMERE

Fig. 4. — *The functional metamere.*

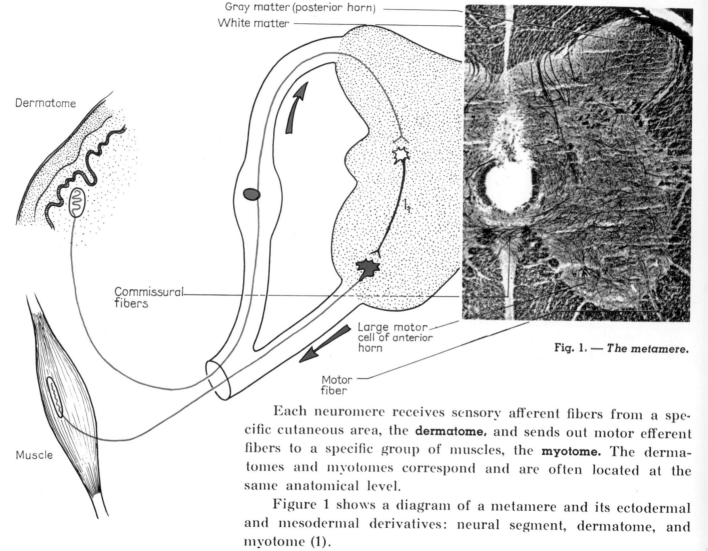

Gray matter (posterior horn)
White matter
Dermatome
Commissural fibers
Large motor cell of anterior horn
Motor fiber
Muscle

Fig. 1. — *The metamere.*

Each neuromere receives sensory afferent fibers from a specific cutaneous area, the **dermatome**, and sends out motor efferent fibers to a specific group of muscles, the **myotome**. The dermatomes and myotomes correspond and are often located at the same anatomical level.

Figure 1 shows a diagram of a metamere and its ectodermal and mesodermal derivatives: neural segment, dermatome, and myotome (1).

Afferent sensory nerves also pass to the viscera; response is made through the motor pathways of the autonomic nervous system.

FUNCTIONAL SYNTHESIS

The combination of neuromeres connected to each other on the one hand, and to the brain on the other, forms the spinal cord of vertebrates. Innumerable interneuromeric associations give the spinal cord its unity and coordination. In mammals, and especially in man, these associations and the enormous influence of the brain reduce considerably the autonomy of each metamere.

(1) The various elements of this organization are embryologically interdependent. In particular, normal development of the medullary segment requires normal development of the other two elements. In general, interactions between development of the CNS and that of certain peripheral formations which are directly related to it, appear constant (see p. 33).

METAMERIZATION

In total, the spinal cord is composed of:

1. A series of nerve centers, the gray matter, formed by:

a) Neural cells deriving from neuroblasts:
— somatic and visceral motor neurons, emission centers derived from the basal plates (anterior and lateral horns);
— somatic and visceral sensory neurons, reception centers derived from the alar plates (posterior and lateral horns);
— metameric interneurons I^1;
— cell bodies of neurons of intermetameric association I^2, I^3 . . ., derived from the alar plates and particularly numerous in the posterior horns.

b) The neuroglial cells.

c) Fine nerve fibers, slightly myelinated or unmyelinated, coming from the cells listed.
All these elements develop in the mantle layer.

2. A grouping of pathways of transit or of association, the white matter, formed of myelinated fibers (myelin is white) and consisting of:

a) motor fibers from the brain;

b) sensory fibers from the periphery, coming through the spinal ganglia and ascending toward the brain, and making connections in the posterior horn;

c) axons of intersegmental association neurons.

Bundles of fibers are compressed against each other in the marginal layer. The white matter is thus formed, from the passage of myelinated fibers in this layer.

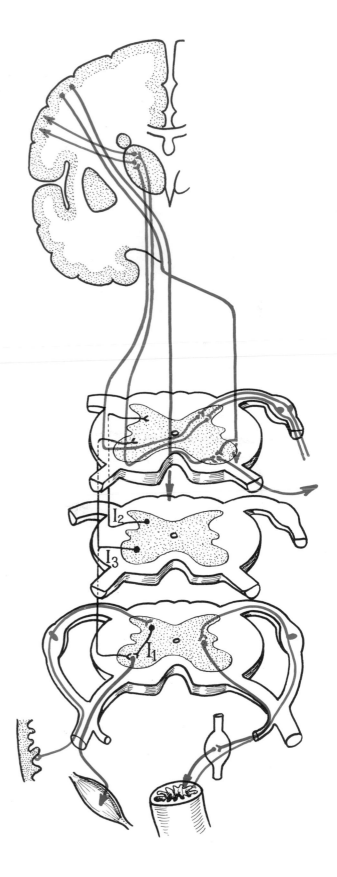

Fig. 2. — *The medullary pathways and their relations with the brain.*
   (*In red :* motor pathways; *in blue :* sensory pathways; *in black :* association pathways.)
   The successive medullary levels, shown differently for greater clarity, are actually similar.

In mammals and in man, segmentation persists in the sensory pathways. It is less well defined in the motor pathways.

I. — SENSORY PATHWAYS

A cutaneous zone, the dermatome, corresponds quite precisely to the sensory root which innervates it. There certain clinical applications of this correspondence:

— In cases of **medullary compression by a tumor,** the level of compression can be determined by the loss of sensitivity in all the subjacent dermatomes.

— In **herpes zoster,** the ganglion level affected can be determined from the cutaneous lesion.

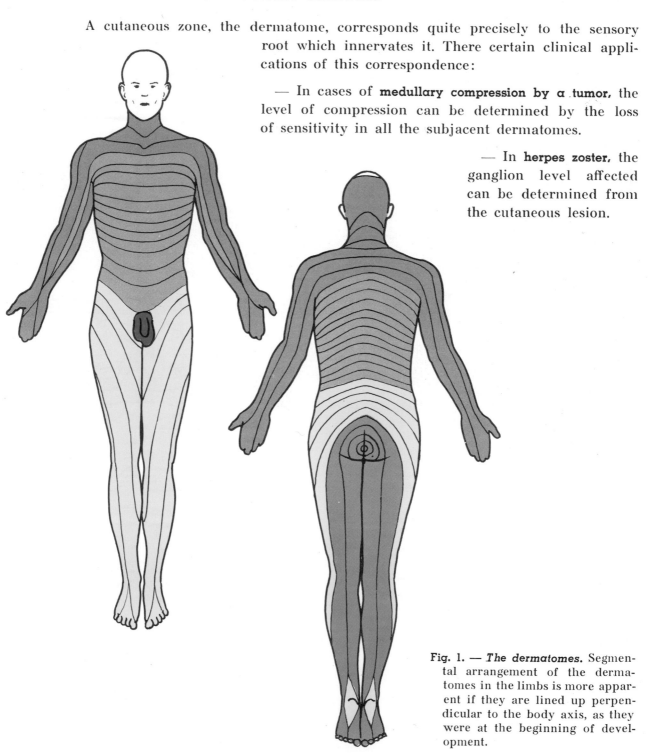

Fig. 1. — *The dermatomes.* Segmental arrangement of the dermatomes in the limbs is more apparent if they are lined up perpendicular to the body axis, as they were at the beginning of development.

SEGMENTATION

II. — MOTOR PATHWAYS

Segmentation persists in the intercostal spaces. It is much less clear in the limbs and the girdles. The primordia of these structures are not located opposite a single metamere, but opposite several. The same muscle group may even be innervated by motor nerves coming from different levels.

Fig. 2 shows the multisegmental division of the innervation of a limb: segmental distribution is diminished or disappears.

In the brain, segmentation is literally telescoped. In vertebrates, especially mammals, cephalization upsets the primitive segmental architecture (see p. 50).

Functionally, segmental medullary activities, such as the osteotendinous or the micturition reflexes are progressively controlled by the higher centers as the evolutionary ladder of the vertebrates is ascended. Thus, man can regulate these activities at will.

III. — INVOLUNTARY PATHWAYS

Segmentation is diminished in the involuntary pathways. As in most of the somatic muscle groups, organs are innervated by nerves from various levels (fig. 3, p. 21).

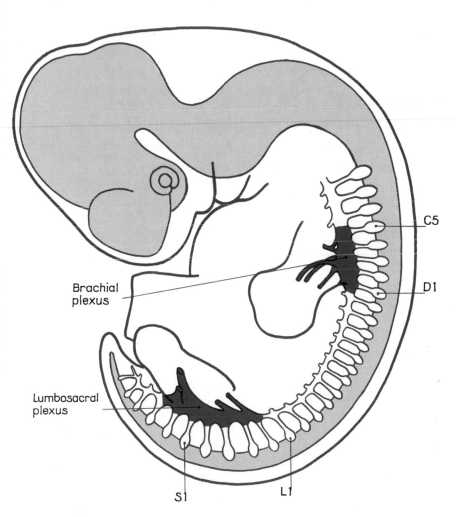

Fig. 2. — *Innervation of limbs.*

Malformations of the spinal cord come about primarily through problems of closure of the neural groove, the causes of which are still obscure. They involve defects in early embryogenesis, since neural groove closure takes place in man between the 21st and the 28th days of gestation.

Formation of the neural tube affects formation of the posterior arch of the vertebra; all anomalies of the tube may produce anomalies of the spine. The most classic form of these malformations is *spina bifida*. Since the posterior arch of one or more vertebrae is not formed, each vertebral body ends with two bony spines framing the spinal cord—hence the term spina bifida (fig. 2a).

Spina bifida is most often localized in the lumbosacral region. When the spinal cord is open from top to bottom, the condition is called *rachischisis*.

I. — MAJOR TYPES

The spinal cord is open. The nervous tissue is in direct continuity with the skin, thus reproducing the general structure of the plate or groove stages of neurulation (see p. 4).

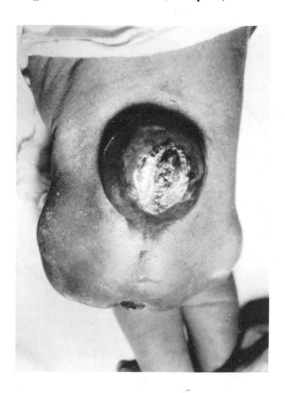

Fig. 1. — *Typical spina bifida seen in the newborn.* Opening of the spinal cord to the skin appears in the center of the ulceration. The mass of nervous tissue is covered by a thin shrivelled skin which blends laterally to the level of normal skin.

SPINAL CORD

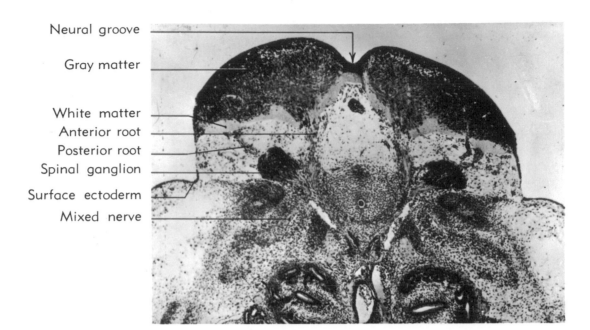

Neural groove

Gray matter

White matter
Anterior root
Posterior root
Spinal ganglion
Surface ectoderm
Mixed nerve

Fig. 2. — *Cross section of spina bifida in a rat fetus of 18 days,* resulting from hypervitaminosis A in the mother (according to GIROUD). A cross section of the spina bifida of fig. 1 would be analogous. Since the neural groove is not closed, the surface ectoderm and nervous tissue are still continuous.

Because the neural tube is not formed, the neural groove proliferates freely on the exterior and the open ependymal cavity allows the cerebrospinal fluid to circulate. On the other hand, the meningeal spaces may be engorged with cerebrospinal fluid, which helps push the nervous tissue outside the level of the epidermis.

Histogenesis is practically normal. The white matter and gray matter can be distinguished, as well as the spinal ganglia and spinal roots. It is the organization of these components which is abnormal.

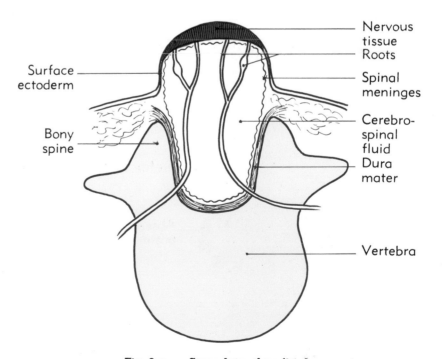

Surface ectoderm

Bony spine

Nervous tissue
Roots
Spinal meninges
Cerebrospinal fluid
Dura mater

Vertebra

Fig. 2 a. — *Stage later than fig. 2.* The bony spines are visible.

I. — MAJOR TYPES
(con't.)

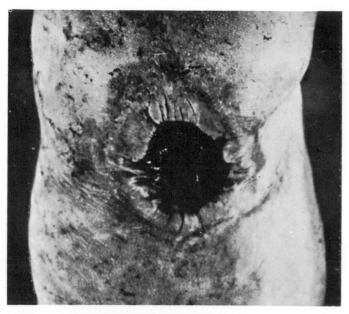

Fig. 1. — Wide and ulcerated spina bifida in a newborn. The dark crater communicates directly with the medullary canal, and is actually the surface thickening of the canal. Risk of infection is maximal.

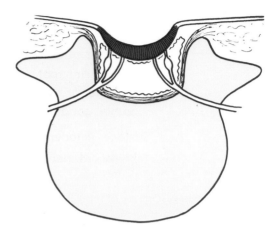

Fig. 1 a. — Cross section at level of lesion shown in figure 1.

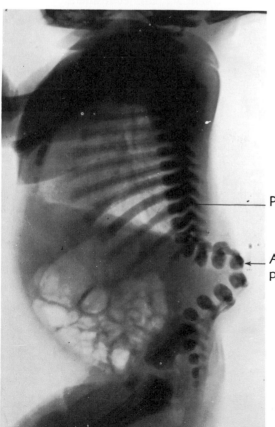

— Profile of posterior arch

← Absence of posterior arch

Spina bifida with " open spinal cord " is accompanied by sensory and motor symptoms (paralysis) which affect the regions at the level of and below the lesion. Surgical cure is difficult or impossible.

Fig. 2. — Here the spina bifida is accompanied by a telescoping of the dorsolumbar vertebrae. Note the complete absence of the posterior arch, as compared with the dorsal vertebrae above.

II. — MINOR OR INAPPARENT TYPES

In these types of spina bifida, the neural tube closes, but only imperfectly. Induction of its posterior portion is defective.

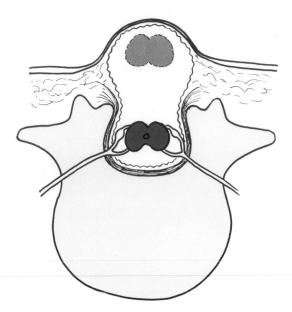

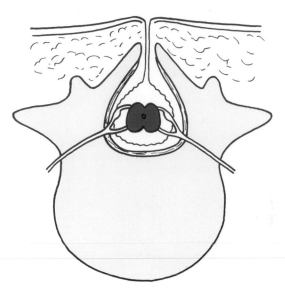

Fig. 3. — *Meningocele. Myelomeningocele.* Accumulation of cerebral spinal fluid in the meningeal spaces produces a meningocele when the hernia contains only meninges. If the cord is also herniated, the condition is called myelomeningocele. The skin forming the pocket is dry and fragile. Surgical correction is possible.

Fig. 4. — *Dermal sinus.* Closure of the levels above the cord is almost complete. Only a narrow opening connecting the meninges and the surface ectoderm opens to the exterior. It may close secondarily.

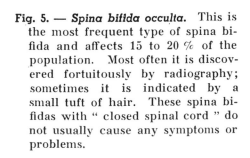

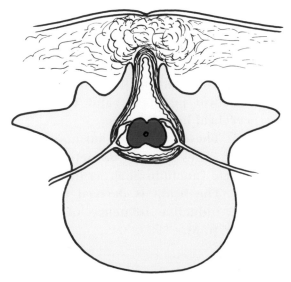

Fig. 5. — *Spina bifida occulta.* This is the most frequent type of spina bifida and affects 15 to 20 % of the population. Most often it is discovered fortuitously by radiography; sometimes it is indicated by a small tuft of hair. These spina bifidas with " closed spinal cord " do not usually cause any symptoms or problems.

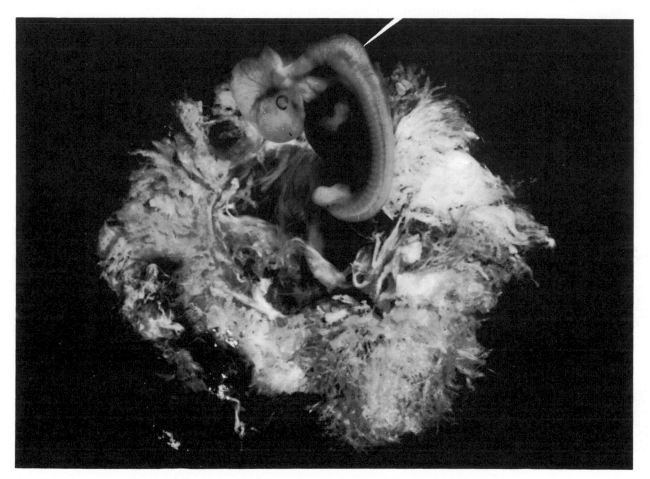

Fig. 1. — *Human embryo of 36 days and its placenta* ($\times$ 6). To the left of the arrow, the brain. The black circle at the anterior end of the brain is the eye primordium. To the right of the arrow are the spinal cord and somites.

The brain includes the medulla oblongata, the cerebellum and the pons, the cerebral peduncles and the corpora quadrigemina, the diencephalon and the cerebral hemispheres.

These structures surmount the spinal cord both anatomically and functionally. They control its activities and can even influence its fundamental metameric functions such as the osteotendinous reflexes.

The brain is derived from the anterior portion of the neural tube under the inductive influence of the anterior mesoderm and the prechordal plate (see p. 8).

OF THE BRAIN

Contrary to what is seen in invertebrates, the sense organs do not determine the genesis of cephalic structure. They nevertheless retain a rather clear influence on its development. Thus, ablation of an eye brings about some atrophy of the optic centers, while grafting of an eye larger than normal results in their hypertrophy. In mammals, nerve fibers from the olfactory epithelium induce formation of the olfactory bulbs. It therefore appears that in man, to some degree at least, normal development of the sense organs is necessary for that of the brain.

During development of the brain, the number and size of derivatives of the alar plate increase considerably, while those of the basal plates undergo a relative decrease. This change in relationships is one of the essential distinctions that can be made between the spinal cord and the brain (fig. 3, p. 53).

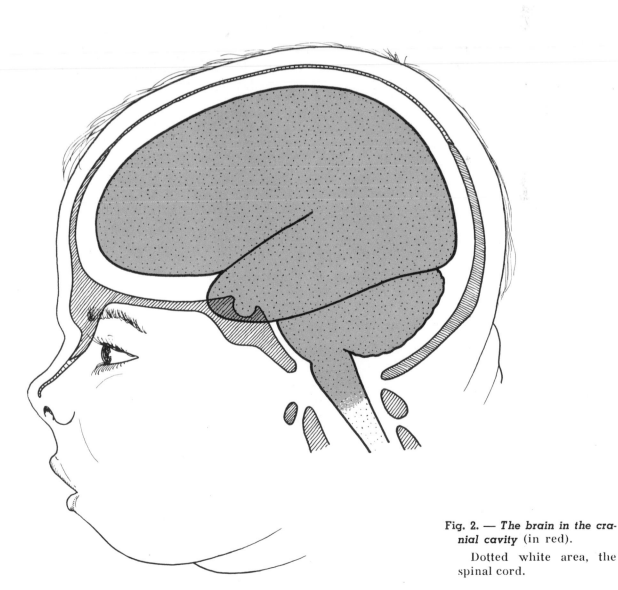

Fig. 2. — *The brain in the cranial cavity* (in red).

Dotted white area, the spinal cord.

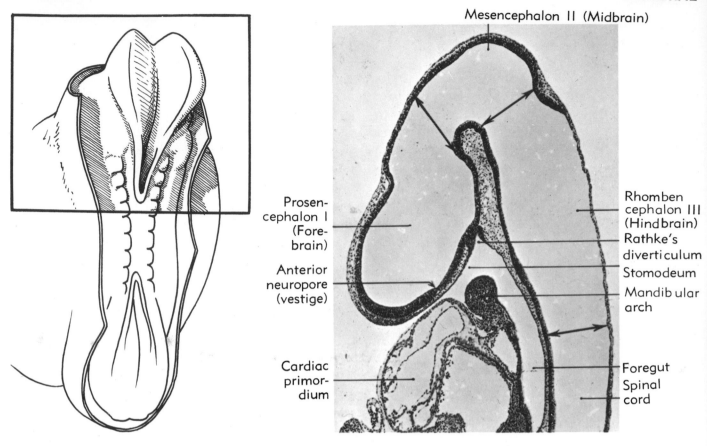

Fig. 1. — *Human embryo about 22 days* (7 somites). The box encloses the cephalic end.

Fig. 3. — *Rat embryo, 12 days* (× 50). Three-vesicle stage : I, II, and III, delimited by the arrows. The first indications of divisions in the prosencephalon and rhombencephalon may be seen.

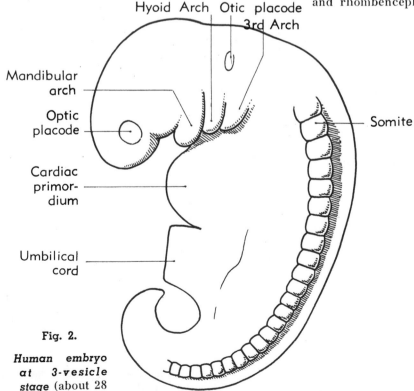

Fig. 2.

Human embryo at 3-vesicle stage (about 28 days).

The neural tube is from the beginning larger anteriorly than posteriorly. Its anterior portion is in fact derived from the cephalic neural plate, which is clearly wider than the medullary plate (fig. 1). Before the 25th day, even while the anterior neuropore is still open, the neural tube enlarges into three vesicles separated by two grooves (fig. 4b). About the 32nd day, the first and last of these three vesicles each subdivide into two parts, while the middle vesicle does not (fig. 4b).

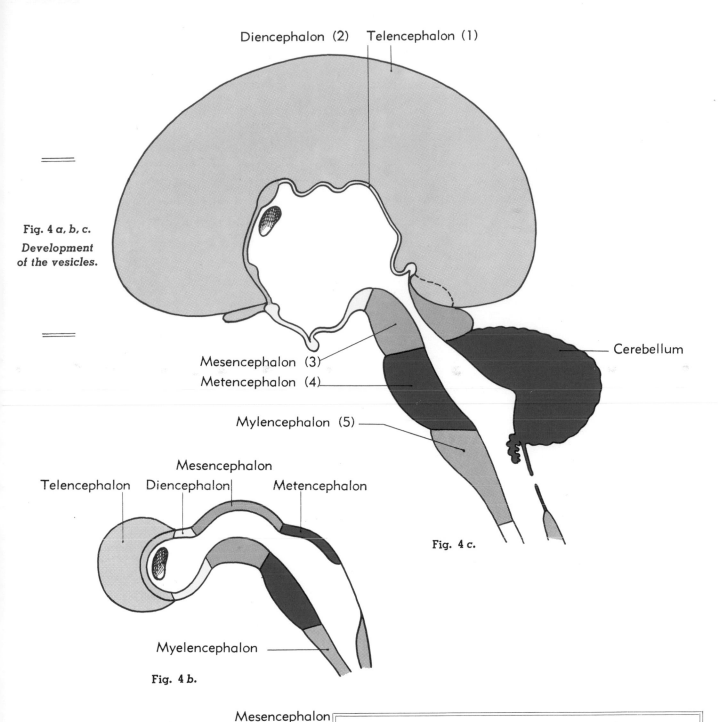

Diencephalon (2) Telencephalon (1)

Fig. 4 a, b, c.
*Development
of the vesicles.*

Mesencephalon (3)
Metencephalon (4)

Mylencephalon (5)

Cerebellum

Fig. 4 c.

Mesencephalon
Telencephalon Diencephalon Metencephalon

Myelencephalon

Fig. 4 b.

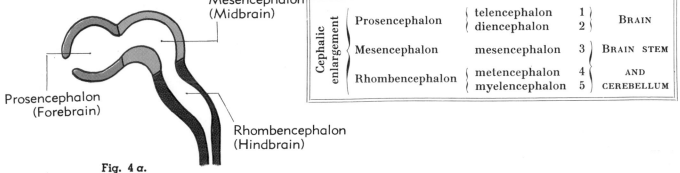

Mesencephalon
(Midbrain)

Prosencephalon
(Forebrain)

Rhombencephalon
(Hindbrain)

Fig. 4 a.

Cephalic enlargement	Prosencephalon	telencephalon	1	BRAIN
		diencephalon	2	
	Mesencephalon	mesencephalon	3	BRAIN STEM
	Rhombencephalon	metencephalon	4	AND
		myelencephalon	5	CEREBELLUM

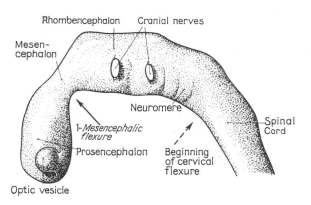

Fig. 1. — *Human embryo of about 28 days* (4 mm). External view.

While the various cerebral vesicles are appearing, the central nervous system increases in size. In higher mammals, especially in man, enormous development of the telencephalic derivatives (the cerebral hemispheres) is the most characteristic phenomenon. The other vesicles, relative to their appearance in lower mammals, undergo less important transformations.

At first, while the anterior neuropore is not yet closed, growth of the dorsal portions of the cephal-

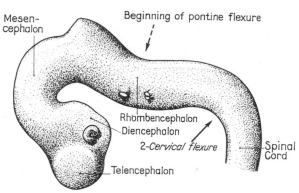

Fig. 2 a.

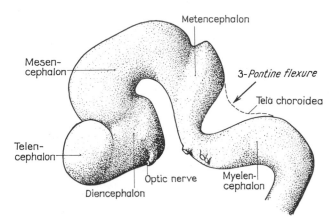

Fig. 3 a.

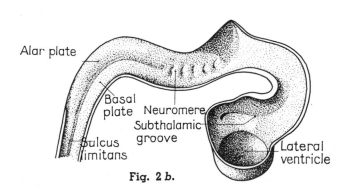

Fig. 2 b.

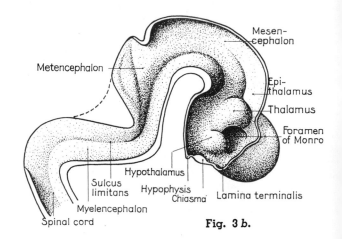

Fig. 3 b.

Fig. 2. — *Human embryo of about 36 days* (9 mm).

a) External view.
b) Sagittal section; internal view.

Fig. 3. — *Human embryo of about 39 days* (11 mm).

a) External view.
b) Sagittal section; internal view.

The diagrams on pp. 36 and 37 are according to HOCHSTETTER and HINES.

AND FLEXURES

ic tube is greater than that of the ventral portions.

This dorsal growth results in the first flexure, the mesencephalic flexure, which appears in the 3-vesicle stage (fig. 1).

Ultimately, the general appearance of the brain is profoundly modified by unequal growth of the vesicles and the appearance of new flexures: cervical (fig. 2a), pontine (fig. 3a), and telencephalic (fig. 6).

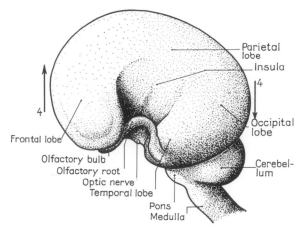

Fig. 6. — *Human embryo of about 4 months* (100 mm).

The arrows numbered 4 show the cephalic flexure, which is much more marked in man than in other mammals.

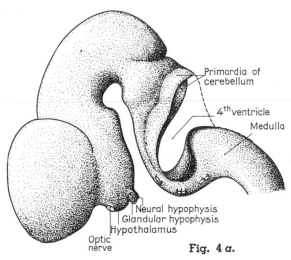

Fig. 4 a.

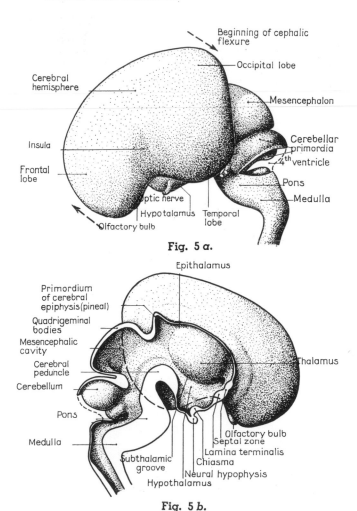

Fig. 5 a.

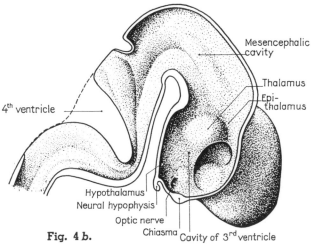

Fig. 4 b.

Fig. 4. — *Human embryo of about 44 days* (15 mm).

a) External view.
b) Sagittal section; internal view.

Fig. 5 b.

Fig. 5. — *Human embryo of about 72 days* (53 mm).

a) External view.
b) Sagittal section; internal view.

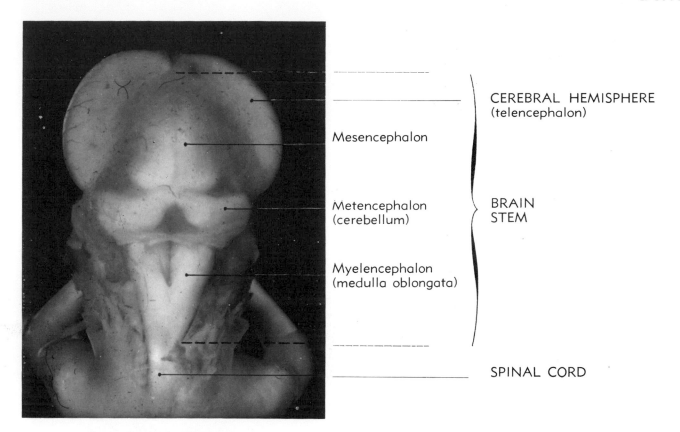

CEREBRAL HEMISPHERE
(telencephalon)

Mesencephalon

Metencephalon
(cerebellum)

BRAIN
STEM

Myelencephalon
(medulla oblongata)

SPINAL CORD

Fig. 1. — *Human fetus of 70 days.*
Posterior aspect (× 5).

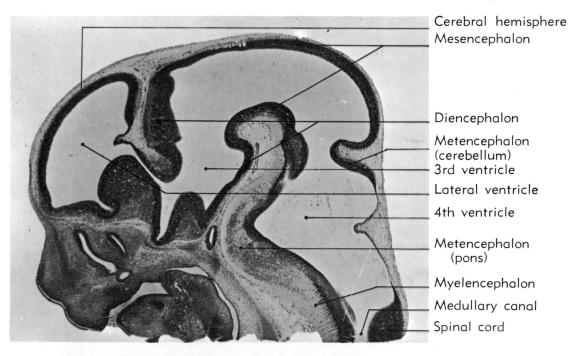

Cerebral hemisphere
Mesencephalon

Diencephalon

Metencephalon
(cerebellum)

3rd ventricle

Lateral ventricle

4th ventricle

Metencephalon
(pons)

Myelencephalon

Medullary canal

Spinal cord

Fig. 2. — *Rat fetus of 15 days* (× 20). Sagittal section.

STEM

The myelencephalon, the metencephalon, and the mesencephalon form the brain stem. The cerebellum is derived from, and attached to, the brain stem. The same structures are found here as in the spinal cord: the alar and basal plates, and the marginal layer. However, their topography is greatly modified. In the brain stem, gray and white matter are not in the same relationship to each other as they are in the spinal cord, and gray matter does not have the same potential. Comparative anatomy and comparative embryology provide an explanation for these changes: cephalization, through which these suprasegmental structures are formed, begins.

Study of the development of each vesicle reveals how these alterations come about. In this development, there is always a roof plate derived from the dorsal portion of the neural tube, and a floor plate derived from its ventral portion. The roof plate, the floor plate, and their lateral boundaries delimit the cavities of the neural tube, the future ventricles or interventricular communications. The myelencephalic cavity, through its caudal extremity, is in communication with the spinal canal and the mesencephalic cavity, and, through its cephalic extremity, with the 3rd ventricle (diencephalon).

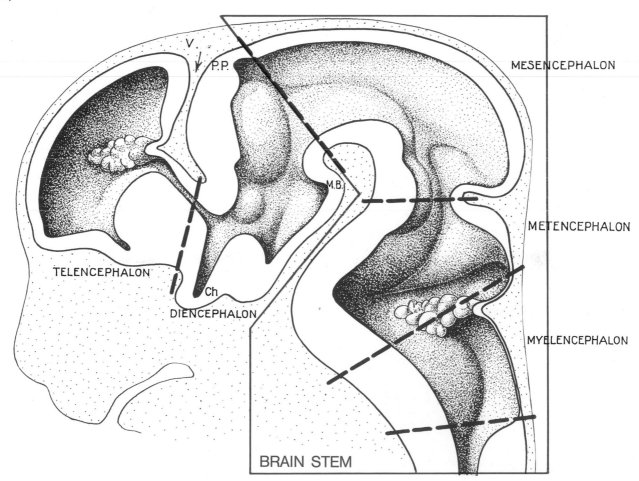

Fig. 3. — *Limits of the various vesicles.*

V : vestige of velum transversum (see p. 53); *Ch :* chiasma;
M.B. : mammillary body; *P.P. :* primordium of pineal body.

At the level of the myelencephalon, the walls of the cephalic tube open like a book: the central cavity enlarges and becomes the 4th ventricle (arrows, fig. 2a).

I. — DEVELOPMENT OF ROOF PLATE

The roof plate, which is very thin because of the lateral stretching, is formed by a single layer of ependymal cells lined on the exterior by a richly vascularized mesenchymal tissue. This arrangement constitutes the tela choroidea of the 4th ventricle (fig. 3).

In some places, the tela infolds forming the choroid plexus, which secretes part of the cerebrospinal fluid (fig. 3). At one point medially, and at two places laterally, the foramen of Magendie and the foramina of Luschka are formed by resorption of the tela choroidea. Here passage of the cerebrospinal fluid from the 4th ventricle into the subarachnoid spaces occurs.

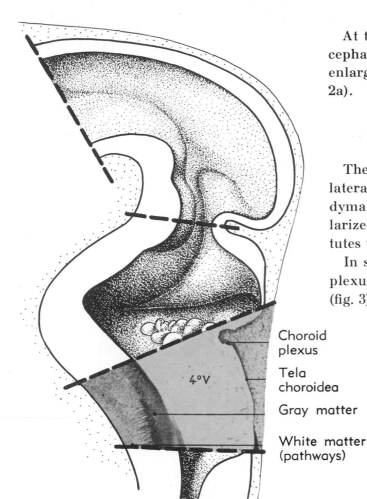

Choroid plexus

Tela choroidea

4°V

Gray matter

White matter (pathways)

Fig. 1. — *The myelencephalon in the brain stem.*
Sagittal section of a 15-day rat fetus.

Choroid plexus

4th ventricle

Fig. 2 a.

Fig. 2 b.

Fig. 2. — *Comparison of structure of spinal cord* (a) *and medulla* (b). In (b), the arrows indicate the cellular migration resulting in the primordia of the olivary nuclei (see fig. 3).

II. — DEVELOPMENT OF LATERAL WALLS AND FLOOR PLATE

The lateral walls and floor plate thicken to form the medulla oblongata. Here the structural elements of the alar and basal plates are everted (see fig. 2b). In the spinal cord, these plates form a macroscopically continuous whole. In the medulla, on the other hand, the fibers of the white matter, now concentrated ventrally by the eversion of the myelencephalon, contribute to the fragmentation of the alar and basal plates (fig. 3).

The roof plate encloses a number of well differentiated nuclei, motor and sensory nuclei related to the cranial nerves; sensory nuclei specific to the medulla (nuclei of Goll, Burdach, and von Monakow) which serve as relay stations for the sensory proprioceptive fibers going to the thalamus and the cerebellum; and autonomic nuclei (fig. 4). These autonomic nuclei affect the entire body; they are the regulatory centers for cardiac, respiratory, and digestive function.

The olivary nucleus, derived from the alar plates, is a relay station on the extrapyramidal motor pathways and the cerebrospinal sensory pathways (fig. 2b, 3, and 4).

The roof plate also encloses the descending motor pathways (coming from the upper centers) and ascending sensory pathways (going to the upper centers) (fig. 1 and 3).

The lateral walls give rise to the inferior cerebellar peduncles including the spinocerebellar, cerebellomedullary, and vestibulocerebellar tracts.

In general, the organization of the medulla is similar to that of the spinal cord, especially in regard to the somatomotor and somatosensory structures. In the medulla, segmentation of neuromeres is even more apparent (fig. 2b, p. 36). However, the medulla shows the suprasegmental characteristics of all brain structures as exemplified in its olivary nucleus and its specific sensory nuclei.

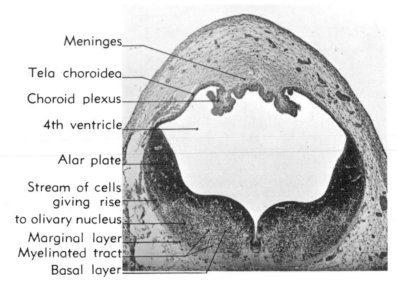

Meninges
Tela choroidea
Choroid plexus
4th ventricle
Alar plate
Stream of cells giving rise to olivary nucleus
Marginal layer
Myelinated tract
Basal layer

Fig. 3. — *Myelencephalon of a human fetus of 45 days.* Cross section ($\times$ 40).

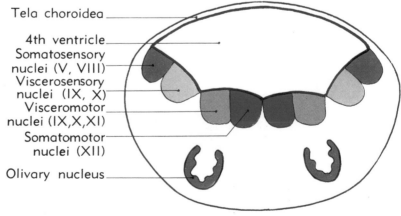

Tela choroidea
4th ventricle
Somatosensory nuclei (V, VIII)
Viscerosensory nuclei (IX, X)
Visceromotor nuclei (IX, X, XI)
Somatomotor nuclei (XII)
Olivary nucleus

Fig. 4.

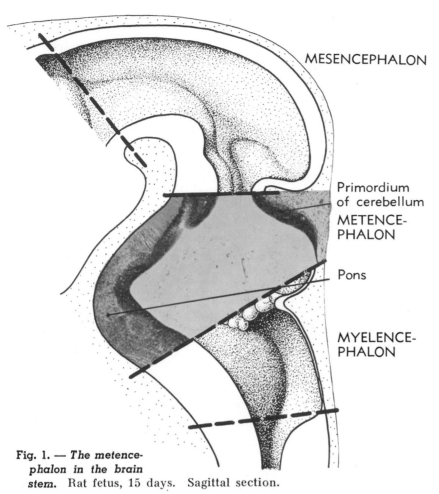

Fig. 1. — *The metencephalon in the brain stem.* Rat fetus, 15 days. Sagittal section.

MESENCEPHALON

Primordium of cerebellum

METENCE-PHALON

Pons

MYELENCE-PHALON

The metencephalon develops at the expense of the cephalic portion of the rhombencephalon. Its floor plate gives rise to the pons, and its roof plate to the cerebellum.

I. — DEVELOPMENT OF THE FLOOR PLATE

Although the lateral walls of the metencephalon approach each other, the general topography remains the same as in the myelencephalon, with the alar and basal plates everted (fig. 2).

The nuclei which are derived from these plates are well differentiated, as in the medulla, and for the same reasons. They are related to the cranial nerves. Their distribution suggests persistence of some neuromere segmentation. However, some of them, such as the V and the VII, pass across the level of the myelencephalon and the metencephalon.

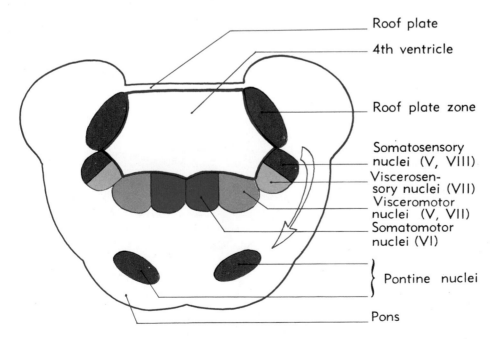

Roof plate

4th ventricle

Roof plate zone

Somatosensory nuclei (V, VIII)
Viscerosensory nuclei (VII)
Visceromotor nuclei (V, VII)
Somatomotor nuclei (VI)

Pontine nuclei

Pons

Fig. 2. — *Diagrammatic cross section of the mesencephalon.* The arrow indicates the alar plate origin of the pontine nuclei.

(4th VESICLE)

The marginal layer thickens considerably. It forms a bridge, the pons Varolii, or pons, through which pass fibers connecting the spinal cord and the cerebral and cerebellar cortices (fig. 3 and 4). Like the olivary nucleus, the nuclei of the pons are derived from the sensory alar plates (fig. 2); they are separated by the fibers passing through the pons. These nuclei form relay stations in the extrapyramidal pathways connecting the telencephalic cortex to the cerebellum. On the lateral surfaces of the floor plate, their axons form the middle cerebellar peduncles.

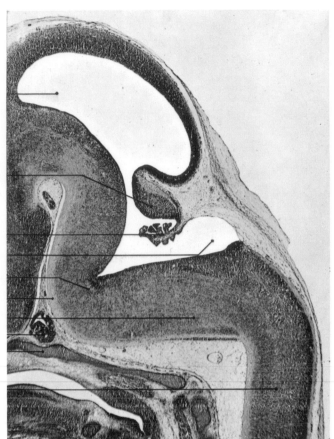

Mesencephalon and its cavity
Primordium of cerebellum
Choroid plexus
4th ventricle
Pons
White matter
Medulla
Hypophysis
Sphenoid
Spinal cord

Fig. 3. — *Rat fetus, 18 days.*
Sagittal section of brain stem (× 21).

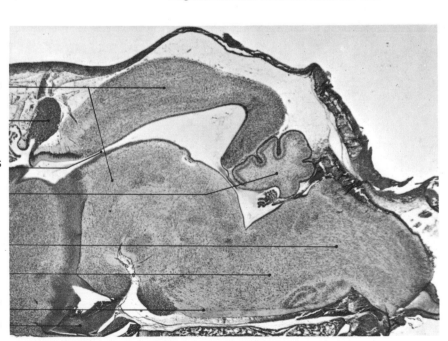

Mesencephalon
Cerebral epiphysis (pineal body)
Aqueduct of Sylvius
Cerebellum
Medulla
Pons (nuclei and fibers)
White matter
Hypophysis

Fig. 4. — *Newborn rat.*
Sagittal section of brain stem (× 19).

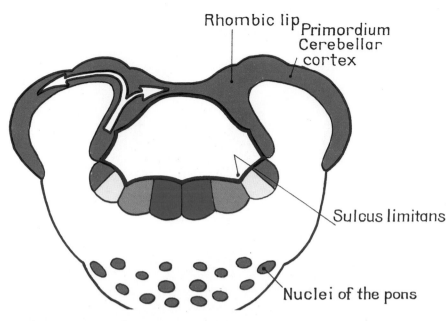

Fig. 1. — *Frontal cup of metencephalon showing cerebellar cortex.*

The roof plate is derived from the dorsal portion of the alar plates. It thickens considerably and forms the cerebellum. The cerebellum is increasingly developed as the scale of vertebrates is ascended.

In man, the cerebellum begins to develop between the 40th and the 45th days. The rhombic lips are widely separated in the caudal portion of the metencephalon, but cephalically they approach each other in the midline to form a transverse thickening (fig. 1 and 2b). This thickening extends to the roof plate, which is originally thin. At the beginning of the 3rd month, there is a midline portion, the vermis, and two bulging lateral masses, the lateral lobes. A transverse fissure, visible on the posterior aspect of these first structures, soon delineates the nodule arising from the vermis, and the flocculus derived from the lateral lobes (fig. 2).

The vermis, nodule, and flocculus form the *paleocerebellum,* considered to be the most primitive region of the cerebellum. It constitutes the entire cerebellum of the lower vertebrates. It is concerned with subconsciously-controlled equilibrium.

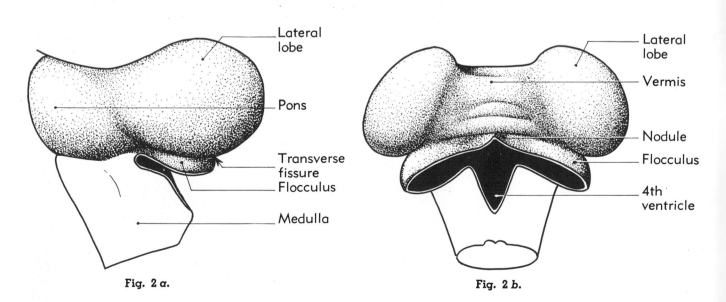

Fig. 2 a.

Fig. 2 b.

Fig. 2. — *Cerebellum of human fetus of 3 1/2 months.* (a) Side view. (b) Posterior view.

ROOF PLATE : THE CEREBELLUM

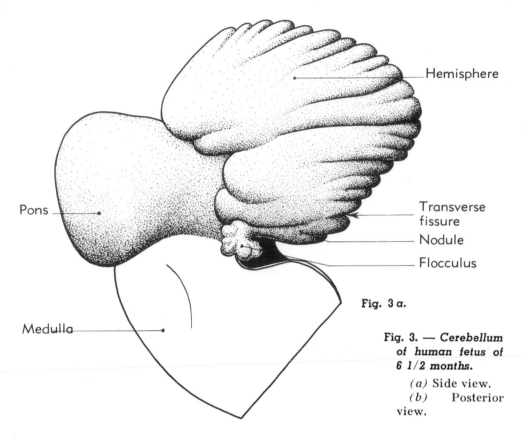

Hemisphere

Pons

Transverse
fissure

Nodule

Flocculus

Medulla

Fig. 3 *a.*

**Fig. 3. — Cerebellum
of human fetus of
6 1/2 months.**

 (a) Side view.
 (b) Posterior
view.

At the end of the 3rd month, growth of the lateral lobes is accentuated. Except for the restricted primitive areas from which the flocculus is derived, the lateral lobes give rise to the cerebellar hemispheres (fig. 3).

The cerebellar hemispheres appear only in the higher vertebrates, and form the neocerebellum. They are particularly well developed in mammals, especially in man. Development of the *neocerebellum* parallels closely that of the cerebral neocortex, with which it is functionally closely related.

Maturation of this system takes place slowly after birth, while that of the paleocerebellum is complete before term.

The lamellar structure of the cerebellar surface appears during the 4th month, first on the vermis, then on the hemispheres (fig. 2 and 3).

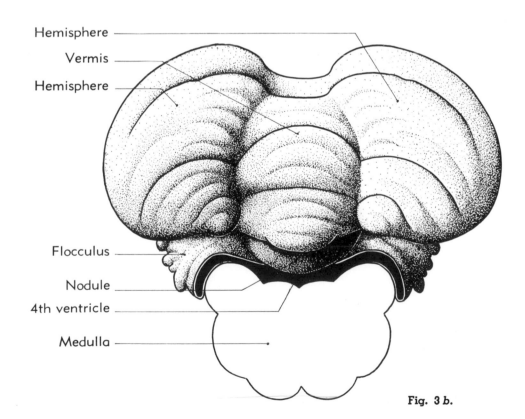

Hemisphere

Vermis

Hemisphere

Flocculus

Nodule

4th ventricle

Medulla

Fig. 3 *b.*

At the junction of the cerebellar primordium and the roof plate of the 4th ventricle, cells coming from the mantle layer migrate toward the surface. They colonize the marginal layer and give rise to a cortical layer (fig. 1 and 1a). They then move to deeper layers to form the granular cells and the Golgi cells, leaving the surface cell-free. This later becomes the molecular layer (fig. 2, 2a, and 3).

Simultaneously, certain cells of the mantle layer, larger than the others, migrate towards the surface and become Purkinje cells. Their dendrites form the major portion of the molecular layer, and their axons connect with the cells of the cerebellar nuclei at a deeper level (fig. 3).

Nonmigrating cells from the mantle layer form the paraventricular cerebellar nuclei. The principal cerebellar nucleus is the dentate nucleus. The axons coming from these nuclei constitute the major portion of the superior cerebellar peduncles (cerebellovestibular and cerebellorubrothalamic tracts).

Cellular migrations are extremely important in the establishment of gray matter peripherally, and white matter centrally, a formation opposite to that of the spinal cord.

Segmentation, still present in the pons, disappears in the cerebellum. Here segmentation is replaced by overall representation of the whole body. The cerebellum can be thought of in this sense as a higher suprasegmentary center.

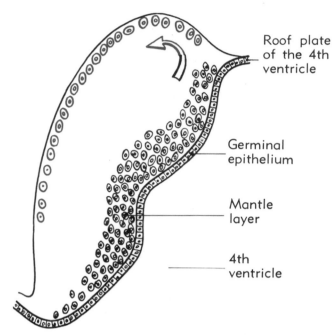

Roof plate of the 4th ventricle

Germinal epithelium

Mantle layer

4th ventricle

Fig. 1. — *Cerebellum of 12-week human fetus.* Sagittal section. In red, the cortical layer.

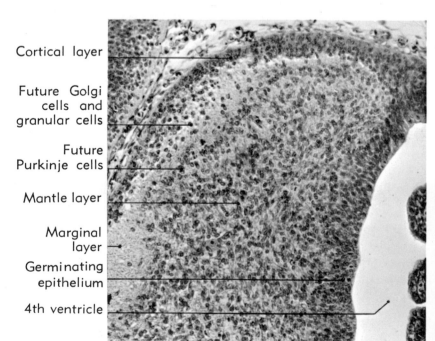

Cortical layer

Future Golgi cells and granular cells

Future Purkinje cells

Mantle layer

Marginal layer

Germinating epithelium

4th ventricle

Fig. 1 a. — *Rat fetus, 15 days.* Sagittal section (× 200). (Corresponds to a human fetus of about 13 weeks.)

OF CEREBELLUM

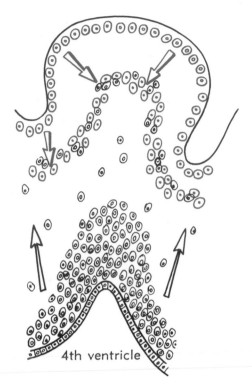

Fig. 2. — *Human fetus of about 15 weeks.* *In red,* future Golgi cells and granular cells. *In black,* future Purkinje cells.

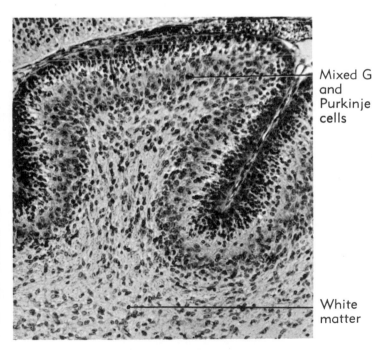

Fig. 2 a. — *Newborn rat.* Corresponds to a human fetus of about 15 weeks (× 200).

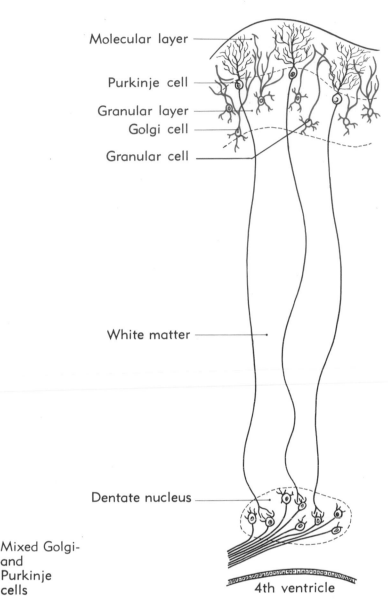

Fig. 3. — *Human fetus of about 24 weeks* (fig. 1, 2 and 3, according to HAMILTON, BOYD, and MOSSMAN).

Maturation of cerebellar systems

Paleocerebellum. — Cerebellovestibular and cerebellomedullary connections are established during fetal life.

Neocerebellum. — In the cerebellar hemispheres, histogenesis and myelinization occur much later. Connections with the cerebral cortex are established slowly after birth.

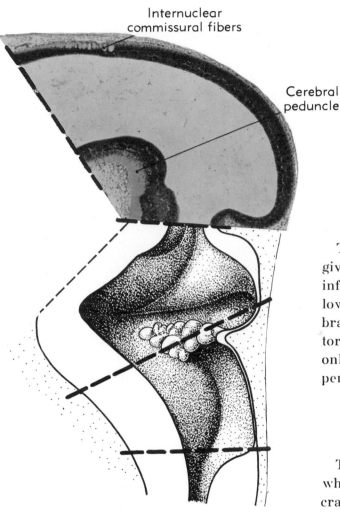

Internuclear
commissural fibers

Cerebral
peduncle

Fig. 1. — *The mesencephalon in the cerebral trunk.* Rat fetus of 15 days. Sagittal section.

The mesencephalic vesicle is the only one which does not divide. The opening-out movement which characterizes the rhombencephalon does not affect the mesencephalon; the alar and basal plates are easily recognizable here (fig. 2a).

I. — DEVELOPMENT OF THE ROOF PLATE

The roof plate corresponds to the alar plates, which give rise to the superior colliculi (optic tracts) and inferior colliculi (auditory tracts) (fig. 2 to 3a). In lower vertebrates, these formations are true sensory brains. In higher vertebrates with a visual and auditory neocortex, these structures regress, becoming only oculo- and auditory-motor reflex centers, independent of conscious perception.

II. — DEVELOPMENT OF THE FLOOR PLATE

The floor plate corresponds to the basal plates which give rise to the motor nuclei of the III and IV cranial nerves. The gray matter of the floor is also formed by the red nucleus (nucleus ruber) and the substantia nigra (fig. 3a). These nuclei are part of the extrapyramidal motor pathways. They come from the alar plates by migration of some of the cells toward the ventral region, or they differentiate *in situ* from the basal plates. The red nucleus has a dual structure, consisting of some large phylogenetically ancient cells and (mostly) new small cells, suggesting also a dual origin.

Facing the basal plates, large motor fiber tracts connecting the cerebral cortex with the subjacent structures thicken considerably the marginal layer. Together they form the cerebral peduncles (fig. 1 and 3a). Ascending sensory fibers pass between the derivatives of the basal plates and the peduncles.

(3rd VESICLE)

The mesencephalic cavity becomes smaller due to the growth of its walls. It forms the aqueduct of Sylvius connecting the 3rd and 4th ventricles (fig. 4, p. 43).

Segmentation is limited to the nuclei of III and IV. The substantia nigra and the red nucleus are suprasegmentary structures.

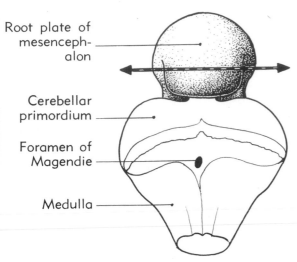

Root plate of mesenceph-alon

Cerebellar primordium

Foramen of Magendie

Medulla

Fig. 2. — *Dorsal view of mesencephalon and rhombencephalon in a human embryo of 2 months.*

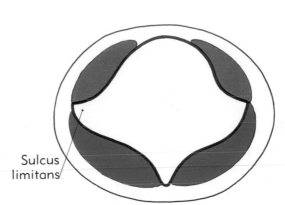

Sulcus limitans

Fig. 2 a. — *Cross section along arrow of figure 2.*

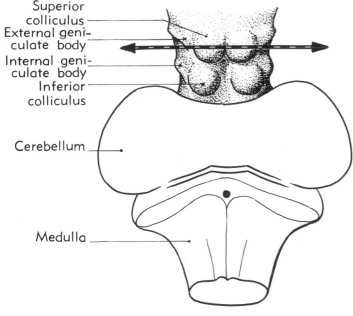

Superior colliculus
External geni-culate body
Internal geni-culate body
Inferior colliculus

Cerebellum

Medulla

Fig. 3. — *Human embryo, 4 months.*

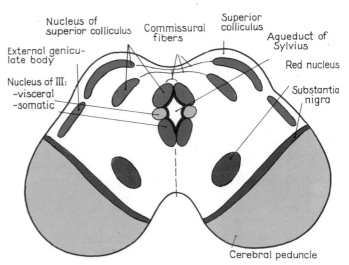

Nucleus of superior colliculus   Commissural fibers   Superior colliculus

External genicu-late body   Aqueduct of Sylvius

Nucleus of III: Red nucleus
-visceral
-somatic   Substantia nigra

Cerebral peduncle

Fig. 3 a. — *Cross section at arrow of figure 3.*

THE CRANIAL NERVES

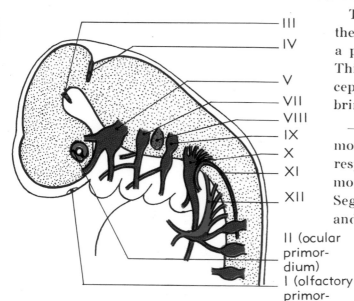

III
IV
V
VII
VIII
IX
X
XI
XII
II (ocular primordium)
I (olfactory primordium)

Fig. 1. — *Human fetus, about 40 days.*

In blue : purely sensory nerves.
In red : purely motor nerves.
In violet : mixed nerves.
The 6th pair of cranial nerves is not visible in this diagram.

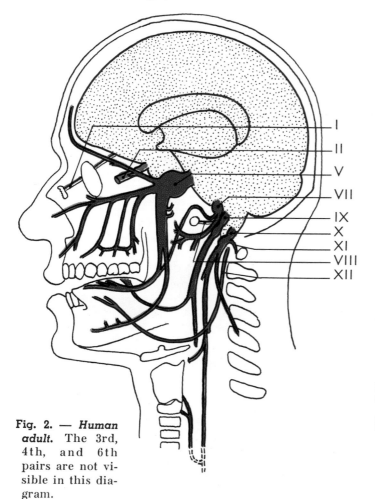

I
II
V
VII
IX
X
XI
VIII
XII

Fig. 2. — *Human adult.* The 3rd, 4th, and 6th pairs are not visible in this diagram.

The nuclei of the cranial nerves arise directly from the gray medullary substance. Since each innervates a precise region, they can be considered segmentary. This characteristic is, however, not very apparent, for cephalization overcomes the metameric structure and brings about two consequences:

— On the one hand, the regions innervated (1) more or less fuse during their development. The corresponding nerves are juxtaposed and often use common sheaths although they come from different levels. Segmentation is thus hidden by complex pathways and overlappings (2) (fig. 1 and 2).

— On the other hand, the cephalic ganglionic primordia do not show the regular metameric division that was seen in the spinal cord. They are divided into 3 cellular layers from the rhombencephalon to the mesencephalon. At the same time, a sensory root does not always correspond to a motor root and the peripheral nerves are not always of the medullary mixed type.

Pure motor or sensory nerves also exist:

— **branchial mixed nerves** (their spinal ganglionic cells come from the cephalic neural crests): 5th, 7th, 9th, 10th, and 11th pairs;

— **purely motor, somatic nerves,** originating from the motor neuroblasts of the cerebral trunk: 3rd, 4th, 6th, and 12th pairs;

— **purely sensory nerves:** 1st, 2nd, and 8th pairs. They do not arise from the neural crests, but from other ectodermal derivatives: the placodes for the olfactory nerve (1st pair) or the auditory nerve (8th pair), the neural tube for the optic nerve (2nd pair). The 1st and 2nd pairs are the only ones which end in the brain itself, without making connections in the cerebral trunk. They have, in addition, a special significance which separates them from the ordinary cranial nerves (see p. 95).

(1) Somite remnants of the head (eye and tongue muscles); branchial elements from which the head and the neck are derived.

(2) This explains why a peripheral nervous lesion can bring about more extensive problems than a nuclear lesion. This is the case, for example, with facial paralysis.

OVERALL VIEW

The derivatives of the 3rd, 4th, and 5th vesicles consist of:

1. Gray matter derived from the alar and basal plates. It includes:

a) **segmental nuclei,** similar to the medullary centers: nuclei of cranial nerves and autonomic nuclei;

b) **suprasegmental structures** indicating cephalization. These structures, relay or association centers, heirarchically head up the spinal cord. Even if they are integrated into a motor system (extrapyramidal pathways), they are derived in whole or in part from the alar plates which even in the spinal cord give rise to the synaptic relay and association centers. This origin corresponds to the role played by the alar plates in cephalization (see p. 33 and fig. 3, p. 53).

Genesis of the suprasegmentary structures is characterized, on the other hand, by cellular migrations which are much more extensive than those in the spinal cord. These migrations increase with the complexity of the organs (cerebellum):

— some of these structures, in each vesicle, are quite discrete: olivary nucleus, nuclei of Goll, Burdach, and von Monakow, nuclei of the pons and cerebellum, red nucleus, substantia nigra, and nuclei of the corpora quadrigemina (or colliculi);

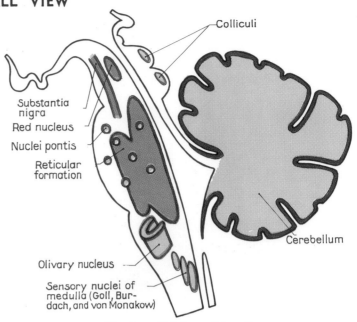

Fig. 3. — *Origin and functions of nuclei of brain stem and cerebellum.*

The inner colors correspond to the origin, the border colors correspond to the function.
Light blue bordered with dark blue : alar derivation; relay center for sensory pathways.
Light blue bordered with red : alar derivation; relay center for motor pathways.
Light blue bordered with violet : alar derivation; relay center for sensory and motor pathways.
Light violet bordered with red : derivative of alar plate and/or alar and basal plates; relay center for motor pathways.
Light violet bordered with dark violet : derivative of alar and/or alar and basal plates; relay centers for motor and sensory pathways.

— others are diffuse, such as the reticular formation which will occupy the ventral portion of the three vesicles. This substance is formed from many small nuclei, and is derived from the alar or basal plates, or both, in variable proportions. Its mesencephalic fraction activates the extrapyramidal motor tracts. Its pontine-medullar fraction activates the ascending sensory tracts and inhibits the pyramidal motor tracts.

2. White matter formed from myelinated tracts thickening the marginal layer ventrally or passing through the gray nuclei:

a) **Segmentary association tracts,** which make the brain stem a functionally homogeneous whole, and connect it to its subjacent and suprajacent structures.

b) **Cerebromedullary or medullocerebral pathways,** which use the brain stem only as a crossover (e.g., the pyramidal tract, the spinothalamic pathway of pain and heat) or which make connections at the level of its suprasegmentary centers (e.g., the extrapyramidal pathways, the spinobulbothalamic pathway of proprioception).

c) **Brain stem pathways** (e.g., the geniculate tract, connecting the cerebral cortex to the nuclei of the cranial nerves).

d) **Spinocerebellar pathways** (e.g., Flechsig's tract of deep unconscious sensory perception).

THE BRAIN

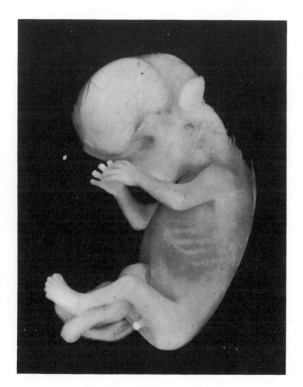

Fig. 1. — *Human embryo,*
about 70 days (5 cm), (× 1.5).

Above the brain stem, derivatives of the prosencephalic, diencephalic, and telencephalic vesicles form the brain itself.

Relative to the subjacent structures, the prosencephalon is characterized by considerable growth of the alar plates and relative regression of the basal plates. Some authorities even believe that the vesicle consists only of the alar plates. Because of this extension of the alar plates, the prosencephalon will produce more receptor and associative, than motor, structures. At the same time, neural segmentation is effaced. The simple reflex arc of the spinal cord no longer exists at this level.

Because of its enormous development, the telencephalon progressively surrounds the diencephalic vesicle, which is encircled by the hemispheres at about 2 1/2 months (see p. 65). Sutures appear between the walls of the two vesicles, thus producing anatomic unity. Only the posterior portion of the diencephalon remains free in continuity with the mesencephalon.

The telencephalon and diencephalon are originally separated by a plane which passes anterior to the optic chiasma, cuts the foramina of Monro and follows the dorsal groove separating the two vesicles (velum transversum). The junction of the diencephalon and mesencephalon is posterior to the mammillary bodies and to the pineal body (fig. 2).

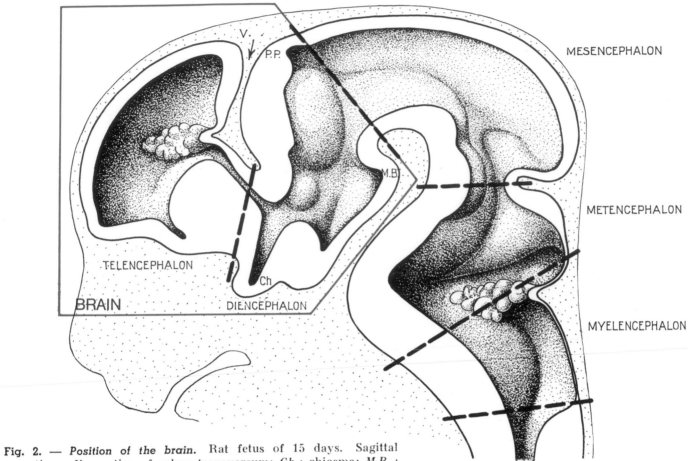

Fig. 2. — *Position of the brain.* Rat fetus of 15 days. Sagittal section. *V :* vestige of velum transversum; *Ch :* chiasma; *M.B. :* mammillary body; *P.P. :* pineal primordium.

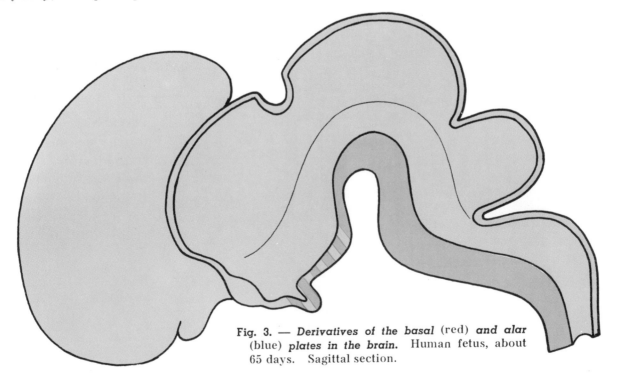

Fig. 3. — *Derivatives of the basal* (red) *and alar* (blue) *plates in the brain.* Human fetus, about 65 days. Sagittal section.

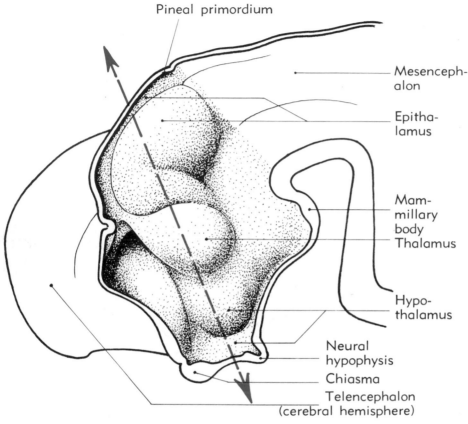

Pineal primordium

Mesenceph-alon

Epitha-lamus

Mam-millary body

Thalamus

Hypo-thalamus

Neural hypophysis

Chiasma

Telencephalon (cerebral hemisphere)

Fig. 1. — *Right half of diencephalon of a human embryo of about 48 days* (19 mm). The arrow shows the plane of section of figure 2 *b*.

As a result of its prosence-phalic origin, the ***diencephalon*** contains many more *receptor* and *coordinating* structures than *effector* nuclei. These characteristics are constant throughout the vertebrates.

I. — DERIVATIVES OF ALAR PLATES

1. Dorsal derivatives (epi-thalamus) form the roof plate of the vesicle (fig. 1 and 2b). They are very developed in the lower vertebrates where they give rise to a large pineal body, a neurosensory receptor and secretory organ. In reptiles, dorsal derivatives bring about a true sensory differentiation, the pineal eye (fig. 3). In mam-mals, the importance of the epi-thalamus is diminished and the earlier structures disappear or regress (fig. 3).

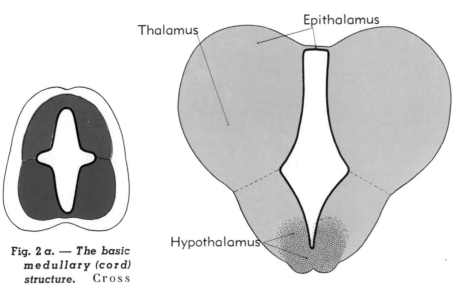

Thalamus

Epithalamus

Hypothalamus

Fig. 2 a. — *The basic medullary (cord) structure.* Cross section.

Fig. 2 b. — *The diencephalon.*

(2nd VESICLE)

2. **Lateral derivatives** give rise to:

a) **The thalamus.** — In contrast to the epithalamus, the thalamus is important during evolution. It begins as a simple relay station in the opticomesencephalic pathways. (For this reason it is sometimes called the optic layer.) Gradually it becomes a polysensorial connection, interposed between the sensory receptors and the cerebral cortex, the seat of conscious perception (fig. 3). Its role is most important in man.

b) **The hypothalamus,** coordinating and effector receptor center of autonomic function in all vertebrates.

3. **Ventral derivatives** develop from the floor of the diencephalic vesicle. In all vertebrates, the floor plate gives rise to the sensory primordium of the eye and the neural hypophysis. In fish, it also produces an organ sensitive to pressure.

II. — DERIVATIVES OF THE BASAL PLATES: EFFECTOR HYPOTHALAMUS

Because of the effector pathways which it contains, especially toward the neurohypophysis and the brain stem, it was thought that the hypothalamus could be derived from a diencephalic remnant of the basal plate, or from the visceromotor portion of the lateral horn (fig. 2). The subthalamic groove would then be part of the sulcus limitans (fig. 2b, p. 36, and fig. 5b, p. 37).

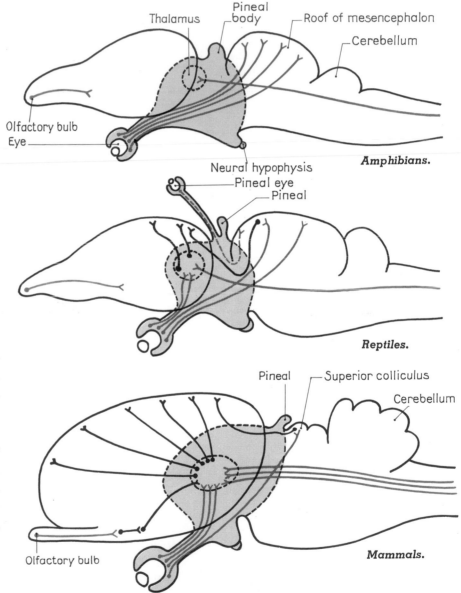

Fig. 3. — *Evolution of diencephalic derivatives, from amphibians to mammals.*

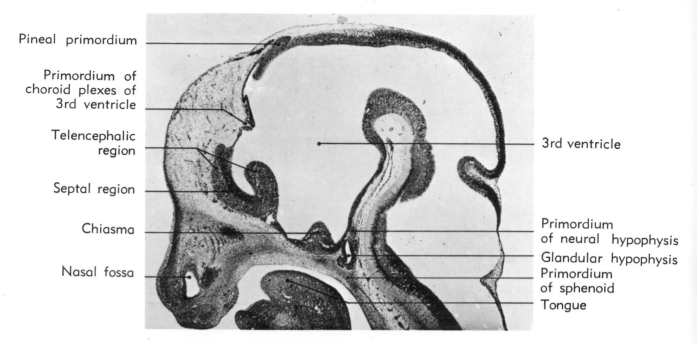

Pineal primordium

Primordium of choroid plexes of 3rd ventricle

Telencephalic region

Septal region

Chiasma

Nasal fossa

3rd ventricle

Primordium of neural hypophysis

Glandular hypophysis

Primordium of sphenoid

Tongue

Fig. 1. — *Rat fetus of 15 days.* Median sagittal section.
The telencephalic hemispheres are on both sides of the figure ($\times$ 22).

1. Development of the roof: the epithalamus

The roof plate becomes considerably thinner. It is formed from a single layer of ependymal cells lined on the exterior with mesenchyme (meninges). It closes the 3rd ventricle above and gives rise to its choroid plexes (fig. 1, 2, 3, and fig. 4 and 5, p. 59).

Laterally, it produces the habenular structures, relay stations between the cerebral cortex and the autonomic structures of the brain stem (fig. 3).

The most posterior portion of the roof plate produces an evagination about the 7th week which later fills in and becomes a solid organ, the **pineal body** (fig. 1, 2, and 3). Its structure is both neural and glandular (physiology, p. 126).

Anteriorly, above the foramina of Monro, a diverticulum sometimes develops which is normally present only in lower vertebrates: the paraphysis. In man, if it persists after birth it can cause small cysts to develop.

Just posterior to the pineal body, a small commissure, the posterior white commissure, connects the paramedian epithalamic nuclei (fig. 3).

2. Development of the floor

Even before the forebrain is closed, the floor of the future diencephalon gives rise to the neural primordia of the eye (see p. 98).

A short time later, it flattens itself between these two primordia and becomes funnel-shaped, the infundibulum. The ventral, tapered end later gives rise to the neural lobe of the hypophysis (fig. 1 and 3).

AND FLOOR PLATES

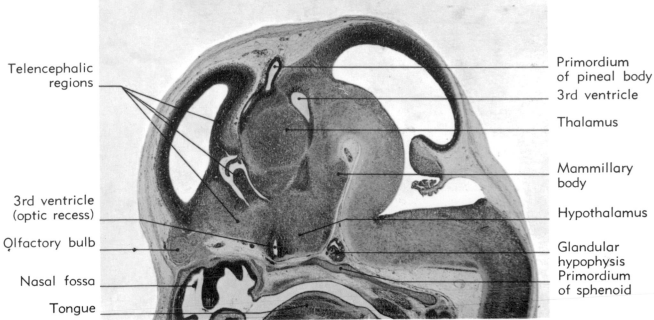

Telencephalic
regions

Primordium
of pineal body

3rd ventricle

Thalamus

Mammillary
body

Hypothalamus

3rd ventricle
(optic recess)

Olfactory bulb

Glandular
hypophysis

Nasal fossa

Primordium
of sphenoid

Tongue

Fig. 2. — *Rat fetus of 18 days.* Paramedian sagittal section cutting into the lateral walls of the diencephalon and the telencephalon (× 17) (see also fig. 4 *b* and 5 *b*, p. 37).

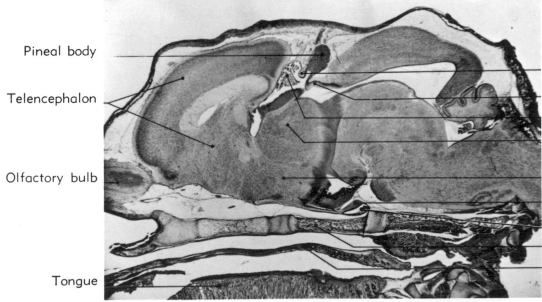

Pineal body

Telencephalon

Olfactory bulb

Tongue

Interhabenular
commissure

Posterior white
commissure

Choroid plexus
of 3rd ventricle

Thalamus

Hypothalamus

Neural hypophysis

Glandular
hypophysis

Sphenoid

Palatine mucosa
peeled
away from the
bone (artifact)

Fig. 3. — *Newborn rat (21st day).* Paramedian sagittal section (× 13).

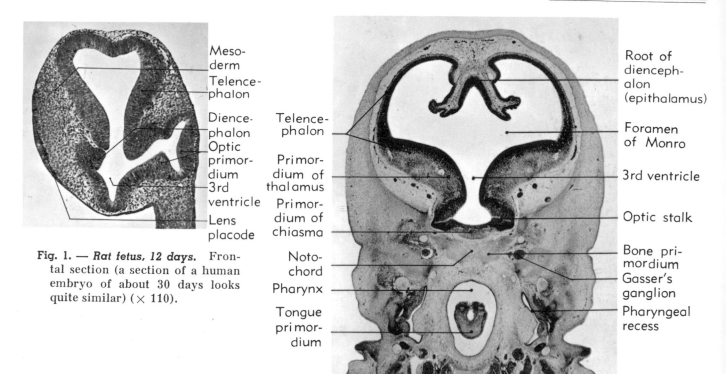

Fig. 1. — *Rat fetus, 12 days.* Frontal section (a section of a human embryo of about 30 days looks quite similar) (× 110).

Fig. 3. — *Human embryo of about 50 days* (20 mm). Frontal section at level of chiasma (× 15).

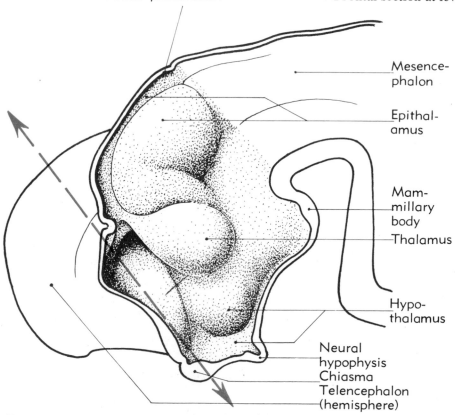

Fig. 2. — *Right half of diencephalon of a human embryo of about 48 days.* The arrow shows the plane of section of figure 3. The plane of section of figures 4 and 5 is posterior to this arrow.

The lateral walls thicken considerably. Their superior portion gives rise to the thalamus, and their inferior, thinner portion, to the hypothalamus. These two structures are separated by the subthalamic groove (fig. 5).

1. The thalamus is derived from the alar plates. It differentiates into several zones which relate it to:

— the telencephalic striated nuclei (the optostriate system, essentially subcortical);

— the general sensory pathways, which connect there before reaching the somesthetic cortex of the ascending parietal;

— the cortex in general (cortico-diencephalic relations).

Growth of the right and left thalamic masses is such that the thalamus fuses on the median line, forming an intraventricular bridge.

Behind the posterior pole of the thalamus (pulvinar), the lateral walls give rise to the external and internal geniculate bodies (fig. 3, p. 49). These structures connect the visual and auditory pathways before their arrival in the telencephalic cortex.

2. **The hypothalamus** (fig. 2) is differentiated from the alar region below the thalamus and perhaps also from the regressive basal plate (fig. 2b, p. 54). It contains various autonomic nuclei which control the sympathetic and parasympathetic medullary systems. Their multiple functions involve sleep, digestion, thermal regulation, emotional reactions, etc.

Behind and ventrally, the mammillary bodies can be seen. These structures connect the hypothalamus to the higher centers of the rhinencephalon and to the lower centers of the brain stem.

Significance of the hypothalamus. — At the level of the rhinencephalon (a telencephalic derivative), there is a cortical region, *Ammon's horn,* which is closely related to the hypothalamus. It integrates the involuntary system and behavior. This hypothalamocortical combination coordinates afferent nerves. The responses it provides are transmitted by nervous pathways toward the motor centers of the brain stem, invoking neurosecretory control of the hypophysis (see p. 125). They assure normal involuntary function and participate in homeostasis.

3. **The lateral wall of the diencephalon** also provides the pallidum, the only striated intracerebral structure which has a diencephalic origin (fig. 4).

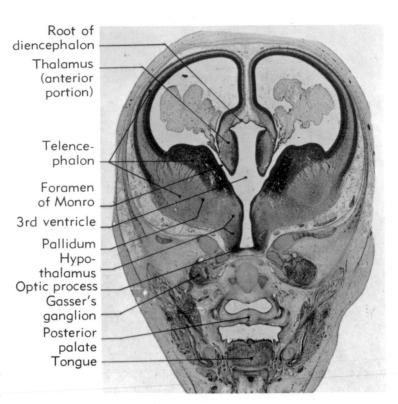

Fig. 4. — *Human embryo, about 65 days* (40 mm). Frontal section anterior to chiasma ($\times$ 6).

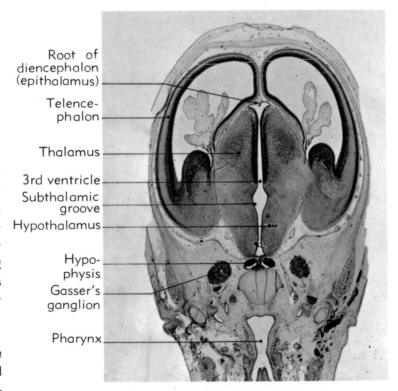

Fig. 5. — *Embryo of about 65 days.* Section posterior to that of figure 3, hypophyseal level ($\times$ 6).

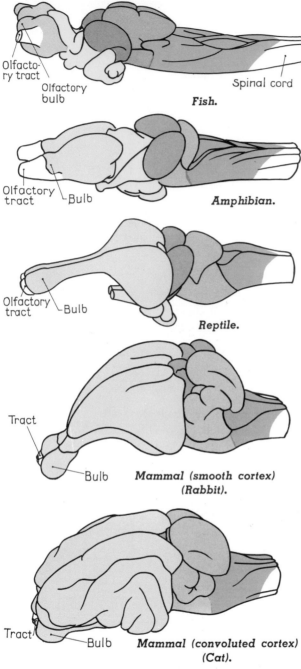

Olfactory tract
Olfactory bulb
Spinal cord
Fish.

Olfactory tract
Bulb
Amphibian.

Olfactory tract
Bulb
Reptile.

Tract
Bulb
Mammal (smooth cortex) (Rabbit).

Tract
Bulb
Mammal (convoluted cortex) (Cat).

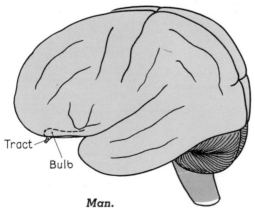

Tract
Bulb
Man.

TELENCEPHALON

PHYLOGENESIS

Development of the telencephalon becomes increasingly extensive as one goes up the evolutionary scale of the vertebrates.

In cyclostomes and fish, the telencephalic vesicle remains simple and its cavity comprises a single ventricle (fig. 1; and fig. 1, p. 62). Only the olfactory bulbs are differentiated.

Beginning with the amphibians, the telencephalon gives rise to two evaginations, the hemispheres, both of which enclose a lateral ventricle (fig. 3, p. 62). Up to the reptiles, this development does not modify the original topography of the 5 vesicles, which are always arranged one behind the other. It is only with the mammals that the hemispheres grow extensively, in a lateral and especially in a caudal direction (fig. 1). Little by little they engulf the diencephalon and surround the dorsal structures of the mesencephalon and part of the metencephalon. During this development, the subjacent centers, which were the most dominant, lose most of their autonomy and are subjected to telencephalic control. At this level, special areas related to the hemispheres are differentiated, such as the neocerebellum, the neorubrum, etc.

Fig. 1. — *Evolution of cephalic vesicles from lower vertebrates to man.*

   — *white* : olfactory tract;
   — *light blue* : bulb and telencephalon;
   — *yellow* : diencephalon;
   — *orange* : mesencephalon;
   — *pink* : metencephalon;
   — *dark blue* : myelencephalon.

(1st VESICLE)

Parallel with the extension of the telencephalon, there is a slow regression of the olfactory bulbs, which are highly developed in the lower vertebrates but are only appendages of the telencephalon in primates (fig. 2).

In the human fetus, the hemispheres extend progressively backwards, following their changes during evolution. Increase in volume and in cortical surface involves mostly the association regions (20% of the cortical surface in the rabbit, 70% in man) and less clearly the effector and purely receptor regions. Progress is thus represented by increased potential for association centers corresponding to the extension of the alar plates.

Growth of surface and of volume is accompanied by more and more accentuated folding of the cerebral surface. Originally smooth in the lower mammals, the most convolutions are found in man (fig. 1).

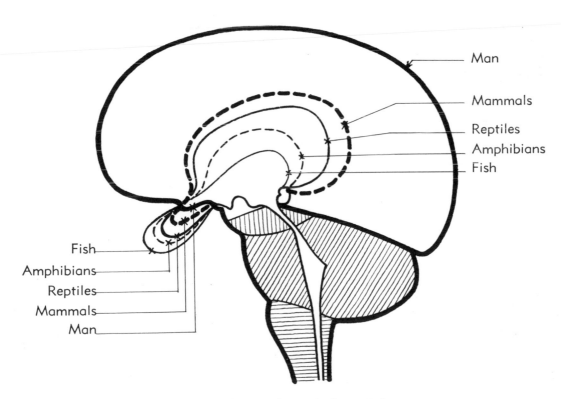

Fig. 2. — *Relative volume of telencephalon and olfactory bulbs in vertebrates.*

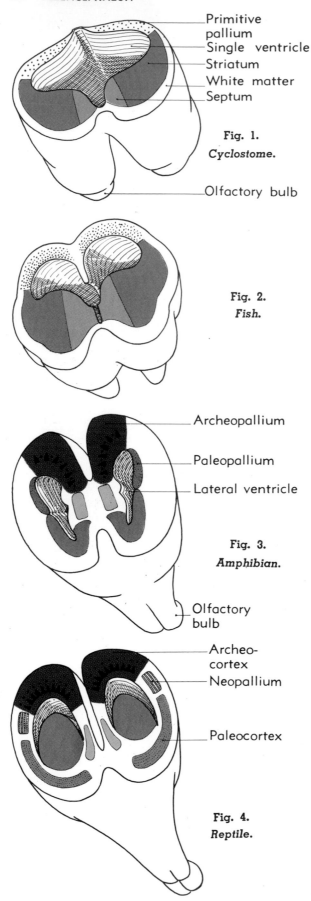

Primitive
pallium
Single ventricle
Striatum
White matter
Septum

Fig. 1.
Cyclostome.

Olfactory bulb

Fig. 2.
Fish.

Archeopallium

Paleopallium

Lateral ventricle

Fig. 3.
Amphibian.

Olfactory
bulb

Archeo-
cortex
Neopallium

Paleocortex

Fig. 4.
Reptile.

The vault of the telencephalon forms the pallium, which produces the cerebral cortex (1). The base gives rise to the septal and striated gray nuclei. The striated nuclei are especially rich in fibers.

In **cyclostomes** (fig. 1), the pallium is represented only by a thin cellular layer without special structure or importance. The cells are paraventricular, recalling the medullary structure. The telencephalon is essentially olfactory and regulates only very rudimentary behavior.

In **fish** (fig. 2), the pallium thickens, but the cells are still paraventricular and do not have a clear-cut organization. The telencephalon is not exclusively olfactory for it receives some nonolfactory afferents by way of the striatum and the septum.

In **amphibians** (fig. 3), the pallial cells migrate toward the surface and begin to differentiate into two cell types:

— small granular receptor cells;
— large effector cells.

Together these form the archeopallium.

A poorly differentiated paleopallial layer begins to form on the external face of the ventricle. It forms a connection between the olfactory afferents and the archeopallium.

In **reptiles** (fig. 4), the two preceding cellular categories are stratified and form the archeocortex. The paleopallial zones migrate toward the surface and present a primitive type of stratification, thus forming the paleocortex. It is especialy rich in receptor and association cells.

The rhinencephalon is composed of archeocortex and paleocortex, striatum and septum. Because it connects numerous afferents, olfactory and visual among others, the rhinencephalon is the center of behavior which although still elementary, is more elaborate than in amphibians.

In some reptiles there is a small region of gray matter of a new type between the archeo- and paleocortex, the neopallium.

(¹) During phylogenetic evolution as well as during ontogeny, the primitive pallium is considered to be the primordium of the cortex.

In **mammals** (fig. 5), the basic innovation in development is the formation of a 6-layered neocortex from the neopallium. This development is accompanied by extensive cellular migrations which establish the gray matter at the periphery and the white matter in the center. The primitive medullary structure is reversed. A basal neostriatum corresponds to the neocortex.

As evolution progresses, the neocortex is extended (arrows, fig. 5). It compresses the archeocortex on the inside and the paleocortex below. This change explains the position of these structures in the higher mammals.

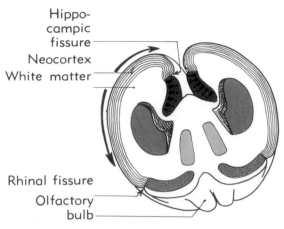

Fig. 5. — *Mammals.*

In **primates,** and especially **in man** (fig. 6), the neocortex is so extensive that it invades most of the former cortices. The human rhinencephalon is thus composed of neocortical zones which integrate it into the new system (see p. 70). Its purely olfactory functions regress.

In the mammals, the rhinencephalon is no longer the principal brain. It is superseded by the " neoencephalon " (neocortex + neostriated structures) on which all the sensory afferents converge.

In contrast to the rhinencephalon, the neoencephalon thus receives a great deal of information. Since it is formed largely of association areas, its potential for integration of the afferent impulses is immense. It is used for thought, and supports activities whose complexity is highest in man.

Fig. 6. — *Man* (according to DELMAS).

At left, connections of the cerebral system in the oldest vertebrates (cyclostome, fish). This system receives only a small part of the sensory information.

At right, the old system is integrated into the new organization, which receives all the sensory information. The archeo- and paleocortical connections are not shown for greater clarity.

    T : thalamus.
    Pa : pallidum (paleostriatum).
    Pu : putamen
    N.C. : caudate nucleus } NEOSTRIATUM.
    C : claustrum

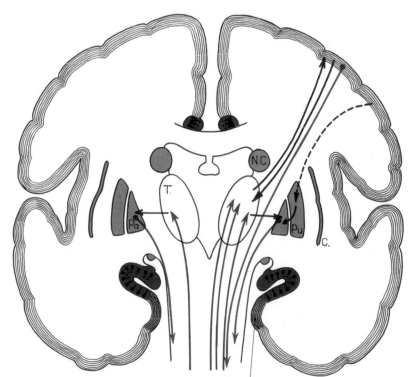

Paleocortex invaded by neocortex

In mammals, the telencephalic vesicle gives rise to two lateral evaginations, which form the cerebral hemispheres. The vault of each hemisphere, or pallium, forms the cortex. The floor gives rise to the striated bodies. Between the two, the telencephalic cavities form the lateral ventricles.

Growth of the hemispheres is simultaneously lateral, longitudinal, and parietal. It is dominated by the enormous development of the neocortex which occupies 11/12 of the cerebral surface in man.

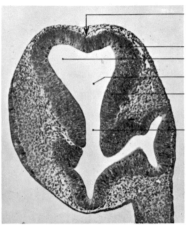
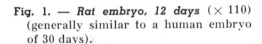

Primordium
of fissure

Pallium
Lateral ventricle
Foramen
of Monro
Floor

3rd ventricle

Fig. 1. — *Rat embryo, 12 days* (× 110) (generally similar to a human embryo of 30 days).

I. — DEVELOPMENT DURING FIRST TWO MONTHS

Human embryo, 30 to 32 days. — Each of the two hemispheric evaginations has a vault, the pallium or future cortex, and a lateroventral region, the floor or future striatum. They limit the primordium of the interhemispheric fissure.

The telencephalic cavities communicate with the diencephalic cavity by wide openings, the foramina of Monro.

Human embryo, 45 to 50 days. — The vault and the floor begin to differentiate. The pallium thickens slightly. Archeo-, paleo-, and neopallial regions, which give rise to the corresponding cortices, may be recognized (fig. 2).

The floor thickens greatly due to the intense activity of its germinating zone. It gives rise to the primordia of the striated nuclei, the lateral striated body on the outside, and the median striated body on the inside. The interconnections of the median striated body with the adjacent diencephalic regions suggest that it is of diencephalic origin (fig. 2).

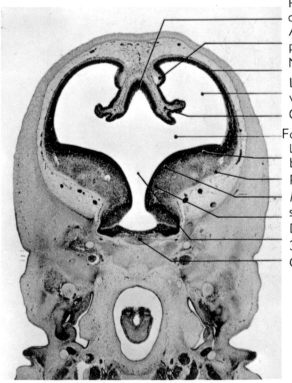

Root of diencephalon
Archeopallium
Neopallium

Lateral
ventricle
Choroid plexus

Foramen of Monro
Lateral striated
body

Paleopallium

Median
striated body
Diencephalon
3rd ventricle
Chiasma

Fig. 2. — *Human embryo of about 50 days.* Frontal section at level of chiasma (× 15).

DEVELOPMENT

The interhemispheric fissure is formed. The junction between the two vaults is thin: along this " choroidal " fissure the choroid plexes invaginate (fig. 2).

Because of parietal growth, the cavities narrow and differentiate. The lateral ventricles, the foramina of Monro, and at the level of the diencephalon, the 3rd ventricle can be recognized (fig. 2 and 3).

After this stage (45-50th day), the neopallium is considerably extended. It engulfs the paleopallium on the ventral side, and the archeopallium on the dorsal side. Thus the telencephalon progressively surrounds the diencephalon (fig. 4).

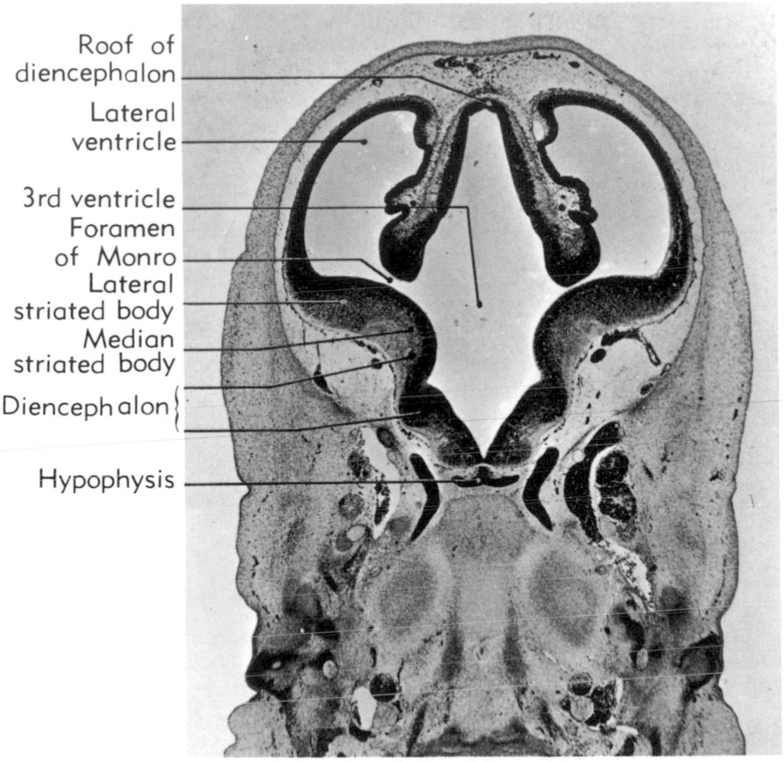

In a parallel way, the various cells of the striatum develop greatly (*black arrow,* fig. 4a). They contribute to the thickening of the area of junction of the telencephalon and the diencephalon. This area permits the two structures to be in complete continuity (fig. 4b). Thus a wide zone is formed which connects the hemispheres to the rest of the neural axis. Fibers coming from the cortex or arriving there group themselves in this zone to form the internal capsule (see following page).

Roof of diencephalon
Lateral ventricle
3rd ventricle
Foramen of Monro
Lateral striated body
Median striated body
Diencephalon
Hypophysis

Fig. 3. — Section posterior to that of figure 2.
Hypophyseal level ($\times$ 15).

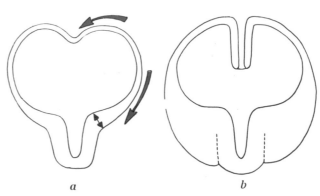

a　　　*b*

Fig. 4.

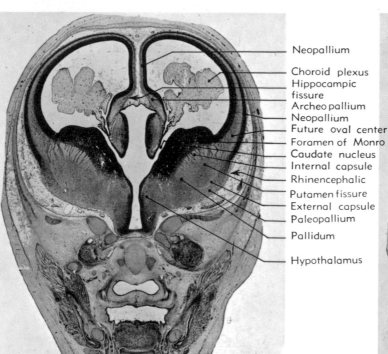

Fig. 1. — *Human embryo of about 65 days.*
Frontal section at level of chiasma (× 6).

Labels (Fig. 1):
Neopallium
Choroid plexus
Hippocampic fissure
Archeopallium
Neopallium
Future oval center
Foramen of Monro
Caudate nucleus
Internal capsule
Rhinencephalic fissure
Putamen
External capsule
Paleopallium
Pallidum
Hypothalamus

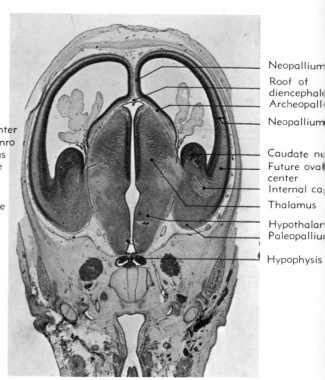

Fig. 2. — *Section posterior to that of figure 1* (hypophyseal level). The telencephalon surrounds the diencephalon (× 6).

Labels (Fig. 2):
Neopallium
Roof of diencephalon
Archeopallium
Neopallium
Caudate nucleus
Future oval center
Internal capsule
Thalamus
Hypothalamus
Paleopallium
Hypophysis

II. — DEVELOPMENT AFTER THE SECOND MONTH

Development of the pallium

The neopallium grows considerably. It compresses the archeopallium on the inside and the paleopallium below. The striated bodies become paramedian. The palleal zones progressively give rise to distinct cellular layers, the primordia of the cortex (fig. 1 and 2).

The parietal growth produces a relative reduction in the volume of the ventricular cavities. The mass of white matter between the cortex, the ventricles and the central gray nuclei also increases. This is the oval center of Vieussens formed of myelinated fibers leaving and arriving in the cortex (fig. 2 and 3).

Development of the floor

Development of the floor is characterized by the appearance of striatal nuclei during the 2nd and 3rd months.

The lateral nucleus striatum gives rise to the neostriatum: the caudate nucleus and putamen. The claustrum may also be derived from it (fig. 1 and 1*b*).

The median nucleus striatum gives rise to the paleostriatum or globus pallidus, which is thus of diencephalic origin (fig. 1). This nucleus is responsible for most of the striodiencephalic connections. It fuses laterally with the putamen to form the lenticular nucleus.

Striated lateral body
Striated median body
Amygdaloid nucleus
Thalamus

Fig. 4 a.

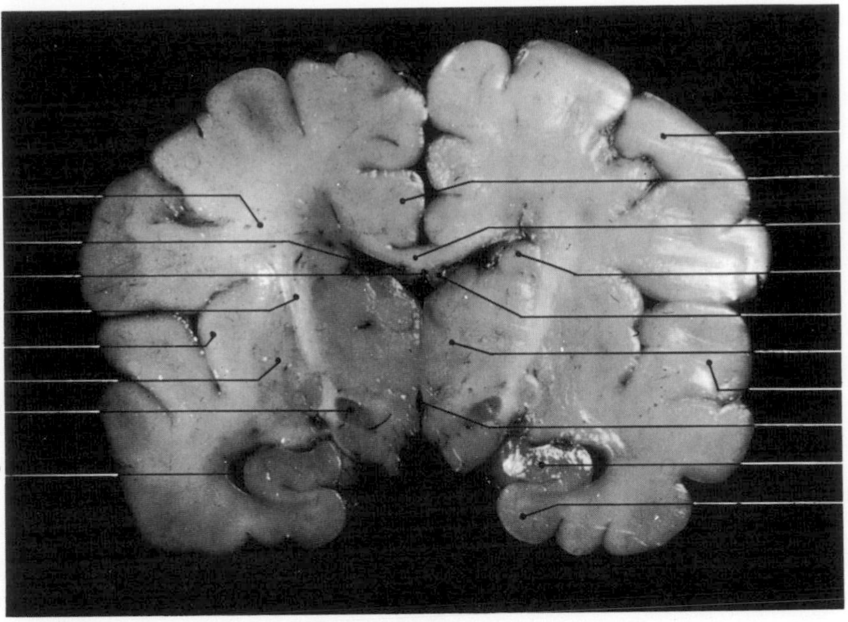

Oval center
Lateral ventricle
Septum lucidum
Internal capsule
Lobe of insula
Putamen
Red nucleus
(cerebral peduncle)
Lateral ventricle

Neocortex (parietal)
Convolution of
corpus callosum
Corpus callosum
Caudate nucleus
Trigonum
Thalamus
Neocortex (temporal)
3rd ventricle
Hippocampus
(archeocortex)
5th temporal

Fig. 3. — *Frontal section of brain of a newborn
passing through the cerebral peduncles.*

The **amygdaloid nucleus or archeostriatum** differentiates from the most ventral region of the floor, below the lenticular nucleus (fig. 4).

During their development, the striatal nuclei are traversed by fibers from the internal and external capsules. This makes their location much more evident (fig. 1 and 4).

Archeo-, paleo-, and neostriatum are closely related to the corresponding cortex and diencephalic structures. The pallidum and the thalamus form the optostriatal system of lower vertebrates without a neocortex. This system is a higher center of integration. In man, it is under neocortical control through the neostriatum which completes the optostriatal combination. It thus retains some functional autonomy within the limits of the subcortical extrapyramidal motor pathways (reflex and associated movements, muscular tone).

The **septal formations** of the lower vertebrates have lost some of their importance in most mammals but are, however, found in man. They are derived from the median telencephalic portions which blend ventrally with the diencephalon (fig. 5b, p. 37). The septal formations form an important junction where the hippocampal, olfactory, and neocortical pathways connect. They send efferent fibers to the hypothalamus and the reflex centers of the brain stem.

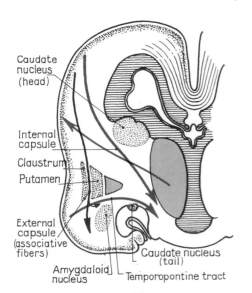

Caudate
nucleus
(head)

Internal
capsule

Claustrum

Putamen

External
capsule
(associative
fibers)

Amygdaloid
nucleus

Caudate nucleus
(tail)

Temporopontine tract

Fig. 4 b.

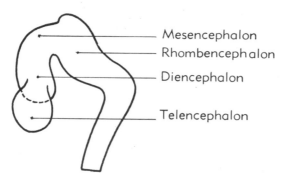

Mesencephalon
Rhombencephalon
Diencephalon
Telencephalon

Fig. 1. — *Human fetus of about 36 days.*

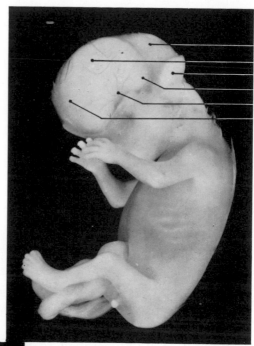

Mesencephalon
Parietal lobe
Cerebellum
Occipital lobe
Fossa of Sylvius
Frontal lobe

Fig. 2. — *Human fetus of about 70 days* (× 1.5).

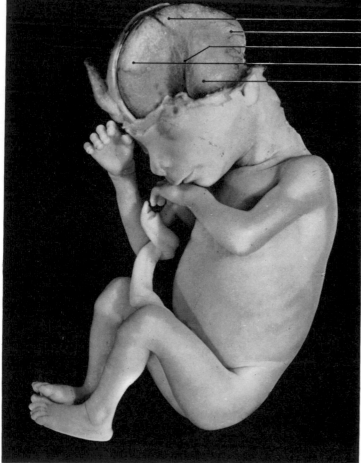

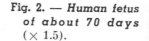

Parietal lobe
Occipital lobe
Fossa of Sylvius
Frontal lobe
Temporal lobe

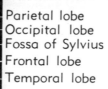

Fig. 3. — *Human fetus of about 5 months* (× 0.8).

The two primitive cortices grow forward producing the frontal lobes, and backward, where they cover the diencephalon and form the parietal and occipital lobes (fig. 1 and 2). Their posterior pole then expands in a forward direction, the future temporal lobe. The center of this apparent rotation is the floor (fig. 3). The vaults of the hemispheres thus take on a horseshoe shape, delimiting a fossa, the fossa of Sylvius. At the bottom of this fossa is the cortex of the insula which develops *in situ*. Because of the thickening of its walls, the fossa shrinks and, about the 9th month, is reduced to a deep cleft, the fissure of Sylvius. In a parallel manner, the posterior areas continue to grow and gradually cover the mesencephalon and part of the metencephalon (fig. 3).

DEVELOPMENT

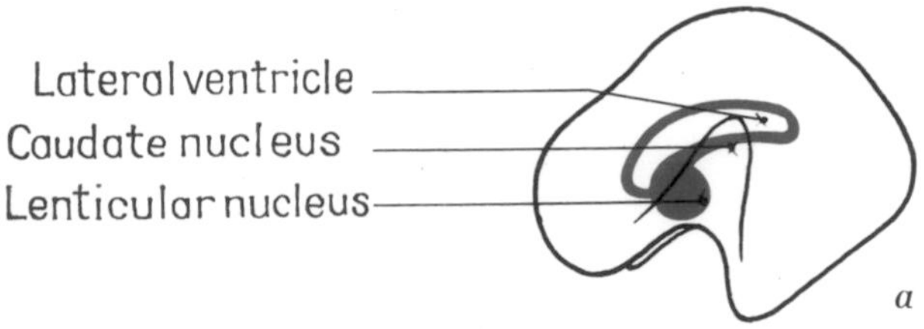

Movement of the pallium affects:

1. **The ventricular cavity:** this sends forth one process into the temporal lobe (inferior horn of the lateral ventricle) and another into the posterior or occipital lobe (posterior horn of the lateral ventricle, fig. 4 and 5).

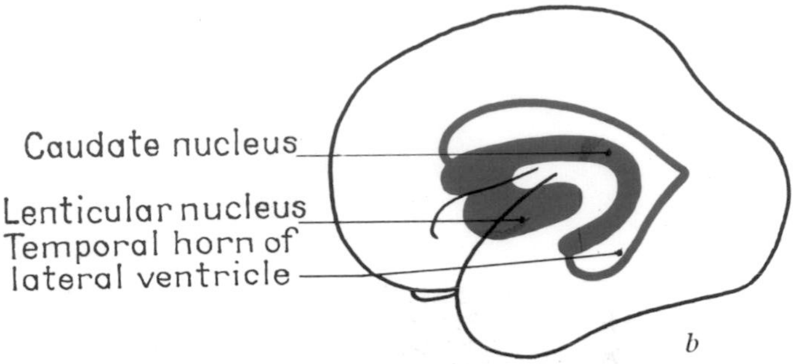

2. **The paraventricular zones of the floor plate:** the caudate nucleus, which protrudes into the cavity of the lateral ventricle, accompanies the turning movement of the posterior pole of the hemisphere. It is thus horseshoe-shaped in front (fig. 4 and 5), and in a frontal section of the brain is represented twice (fig. 4b, p. 67). The putamen, closer to the base, rotates very little. It is simply arched in an anterior-posterior direction, and is progressively surrounded by the caudate nucleus. The central globus pallidus does not move at all.

During its transverse and longitudinal development, the surface of the pallium folds increasingly. Toward the 6th month the fissure of Rolando, then the parieto-occipital fissure, appear. From the 7th month on, grooves form which separate various convolutions well established at birth (fig. 5).

Lateral ventricle

Caudate nucleus

Lenticular nucleus

a

Caudate nucleus

Lenticular nucleus

Temporal horn of lateral ventricle

b

Fig. 4.
*Fetus about 4 months (a)
and 6 months (b).*

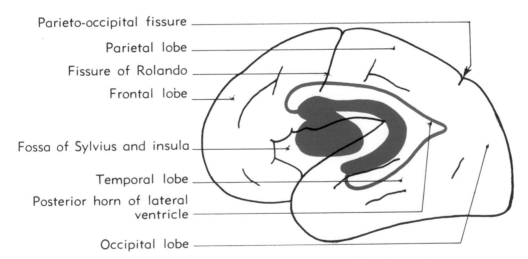

Parieto-occipital fissure

Parietal lobe

Fissure of Rolando

Frontal lobe

Fossa of Sylvius and insula

Temporal lobe

Posterior horn of lateral ventricle

Occipital lobe

Fig. 5. — *Fetus about 8 months.*

The rhinencephalon is derived from the archeo- and paleopallium. It consists of the following intracerabral structures: the limbic lobe and attached structures, and the olfactory bulbs.

1. *Development of the limbic structures*

At about 2 1/2 months, the hemispheric vesicle has a simple form. The archeopallium is found at the internal face of the hemispheres, and the paleopallium at their ventral face, below and outside the striated bodies (fig. 1; see also fig. 2, p. 66).

Between the 3rd and the 5th months, longitudinal and transverse growth of the neocortex, forming the temporal lobe, profoundly modifies the topography of the cortex. Thus, in a frontal section of the brain after the 4th month, the archeocortex appears to be both dorsal and ventral with respect to the ventricular cavities (fig. 1*b'*, *c'*).

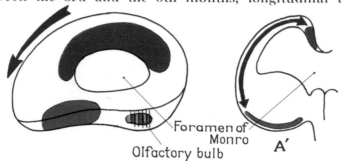

About 2 months and half.

In its growth, the neocortex invades most of the dorsal archeocortex to form the convolution of the corpus callosum, and most of the paleocortex to form the 5th temporal convolution. These two convolutions blend posteriorly to form the limbic lobe (fig. 1). Their structure is intermediate between that of the neocortex and that of the corresponding cortices, except anteriorly where they are directly related to the afferents from the olfactory bulbs. In these regions, they retain an archeocortical or paleocortical organization, and form the olfactory areas of the cortex (fig. 1*c*).

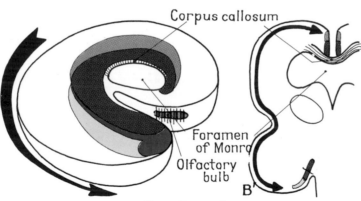

About 5 months.

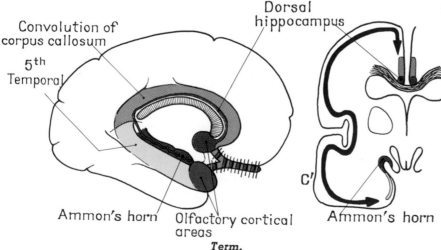

Term.

Fig. 1. — *a, b, c* : right hemispheres of human embryo seen by medial face.

a', b', c' : frontal cuts of each hemispheres.

Dark purple : archeopallium.

Dark blue : paleopallium.

White : neopallium (black arrows show their movements).

The clear purple and clear blue areas translate the progressive invasion of the archeopallium and paleopallium by the neopallium.

THE RHINENCEPHALON

The structures attached to the limbic lobe consist of:

— the intra- or interhemispheric **fiber systems of association** (see p. 74);

— **archeocortical elements** spared by the neocortex, and more or less regressed in man:

— *the dorsal hippocampus*, a thin, atrophied band of gray matter on the surface of the corpus callosum (fig. 1*c* and *c′*),

— *the ventral hippocampus*, more developed, projects into the ventricular lumen and forms Ammon's horn (fig. 1*c* and *c′*).

Through the amygdaloid nucleus, the nuclei of the septum, and the hippocampus, the olfactory areas of the cortex connect with lower structures (hypothalamus, brain stem) and upper structures (neocortex of the limbic lobe, frontal cortex).

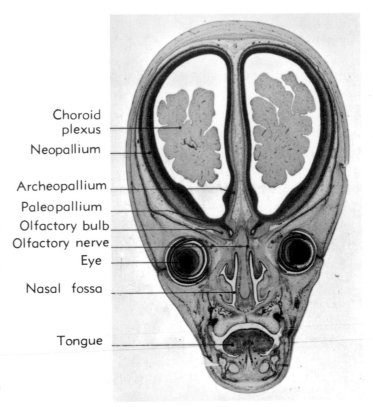

Choroid plexus
Neopallium
Archeopallium
Paleopallium
Olfactory bulb
Olfactory nerve
Eye
Nasal fossa
Tongue

Fig. 2. — *Human fetus of about 65 days.*
Frontal section at level of olfactory bulbs (× 6).

2. *Development of the olfactory bulb*

The olfactory bulb is a cortical formation which develops under the inductive influence of nerve fibers from the olfactory epithelium of the nasal fossae. It is at first a hollow evagination which gradually fills and elongates under the frontal lobe. The enlarged end of this evagination forms the olfactory bulb, and the narrower stem which attaches it to the hemisphere forms the olfactory peduncle. The olfactory bulb connects with the entorhinal paleocortex and the archeocortex of the subcallosal convolution (fig. 2; see also fig. 4, p. 97).

Significance of rhinencephalon

The rhinencephalon is the essentially olfactory brain of the lower vertebrates without a neocortex. It is the center regulating their behavior. In mammals, extension of the neocortex brings about relative regression of the rhinencephalon. This regression is maximal in man and the olfactory functions are reduced. However, the rhinencephalon still regulates fundamental behavior of the species with its neocortical portions.

HISTOGENESIS OF THE CEREBRAL CORTEX

About the end of the 1st month, the telencephalic pallium in the human fetus consists of the germinal layer and the ependymal layer which together form the stratified cellular wall of the neural tube (fig. 1). Toward the end of the 2nd month, when medullary differentiation is already well advanced, the cells migrate toward the surface, forming the mantle layer (fig. 2). The wall of the hemispheres thus has the general primitive structure of the neural axis with the germinal, the mantle, and the marginal (future molecular) layers from interior to exterior (fig. 2).

During the 3rd month, cells from the mantle layer migrate toward the surface and form the cortical layer, which is thin in the archeo- and paleopallial regions (fig. 3 and 4), and thick in the neopallial region (fig. 7). From the cortical layer, various cortical regions differentiate.

— Conforming to phylogenetic evolution, the primordial cortex of olfaction begins first, between the 2nd and 3rd months: hippocampus (archeocortex) and paleocortex. A 3-layered cortex forms in these areas (fig. 5 and 6). The medulla, the cortical region directly connected with the olfactory sensory afferents, has a greatly modified structure.

PRIMITIVE CORTEX

— Differentiation of the neocortex extends from the beginning of the 3rd month to the end of the 6th. It is characterized by extensive cellular migrations which result in the formation of 6 cellular layers. These are first noted at the level of the insula and the parietal zones. (The somesthetic system which ends in the ascending parietal convolution is functional in the fetus very early, before the special senses like sight or hearing.) Cellular migrations then appear at the level of the frontal and occipital zones. About the 6th month, the neurons form their processes, and about the 7th month the various types of cortical

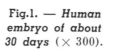

Mesoderm

Ependymal layer

Germinal layer
Ventricular cavity

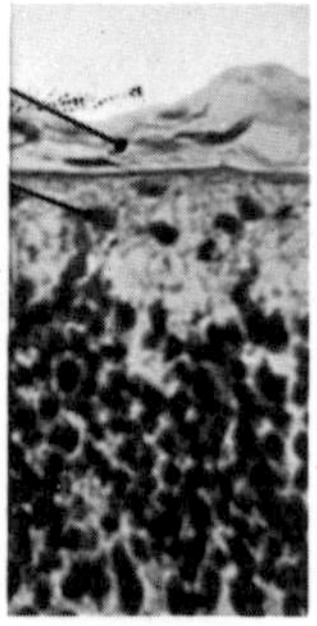

Meninges

Marginal layer

Mantle layer

Ependymal layer

Germinal layer

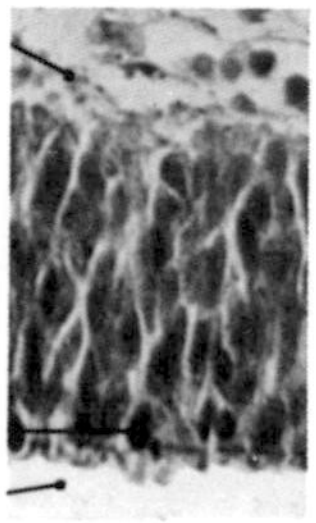

Fig.1. — *Human embryo of about 30 days* ($\times$ 300).

Fig. 2. — *About 50 days* ($\times$ 300).

structures are established (motor, receptor, associative and intermediary, according to the proportion of specialized cells that they contain). There are 80 to 90 in an adult. In contrast to other regions of the nervous system, the germinal layer is active for only several months after birth (1).

NEOCORTEX

The infant is born with most of its cortical neurons: 9 to 14 billion. Only the neuroglial cells continue to multiply actively, thereby spreading the neurons apart. The connections of each neuron increase progressively and reach enormous numbers of the order of 10,000 synapses per cell.

In the adult the cerebral cortex forms a layer of gray matter 3 to 5 mm thick.

(1) The subject of cerebral cortical histogenesis is extremely controversial. This summary attempts to synthesize currently accepted views.

The cellular migrations are increasingly evident as they concern the phylogenetically more recent structures. They are discrete in the spinal cord, notable in the brain stem, important in the cerebellum and the archeocortex, and maximal in the neocortex. Because of their magnitude in these last three structures, the gray matter here is peripheral and the white matter central, opposite to what is seen in the cord (see also fig. 1 and 6, pp. 62-63).

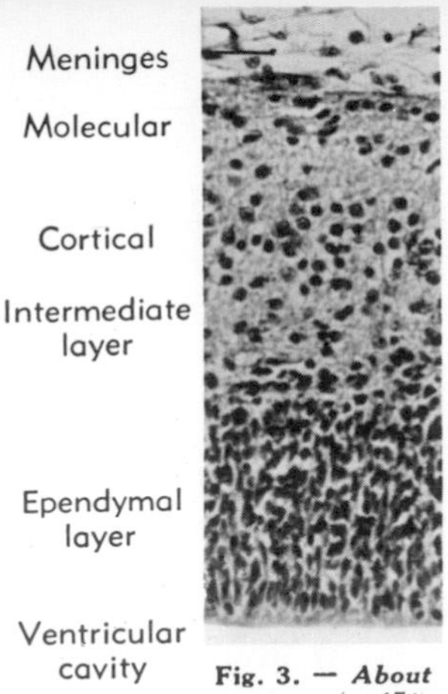

Meninges
Molecular
Cortical
Intermediate layer
Ependymal layer
Ventricular cavity

Fig. 3. — About 65 days (× 170).

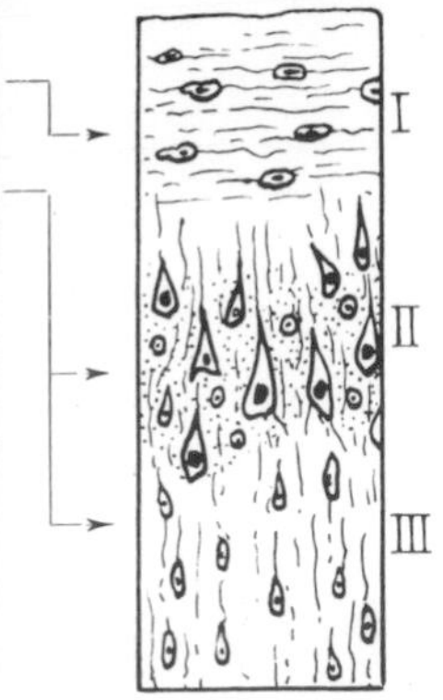

I
II
III

Fig. 5. — About 4 months. Associative cortex (I and III) and motor cortex (II).

ARCHEO

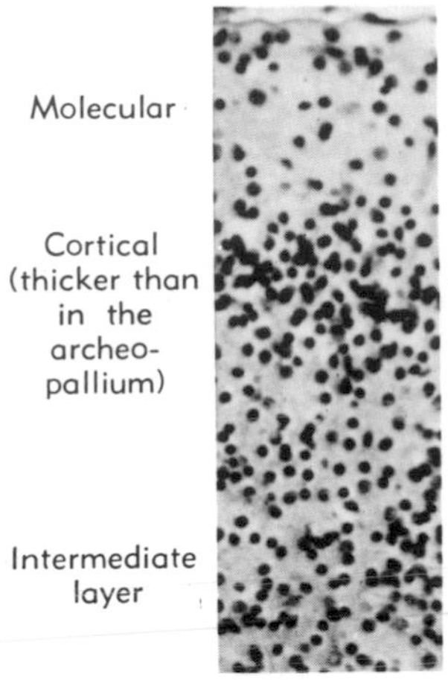

Molecular
Cortical (thicker than in the archeo-pallium)
Intermediate layer

Fig. 4. — 65 days (× 170).

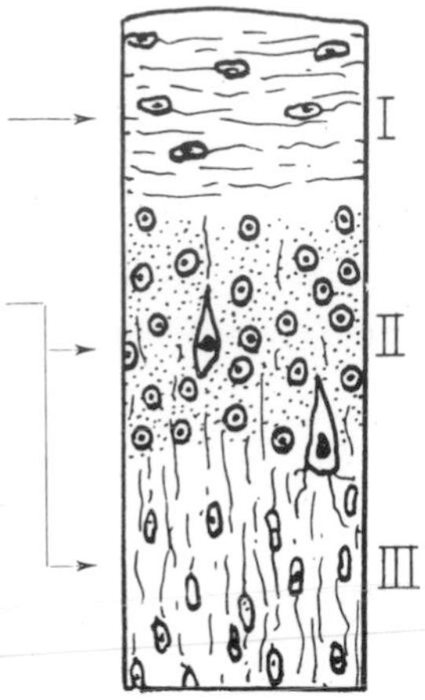

I
II
III

Fig. 6. — About 4 months. Essentially associative cortex (II : very few pyramidals).

PALEO

NEO

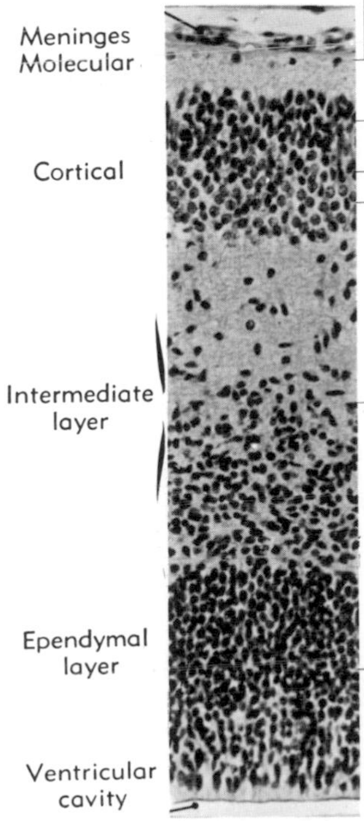

Meninges
Molecular
Cortical
Intermediate layer
Ependymal layer
Ventricular cavity

Fig. 7. — About 65 days (× 170).

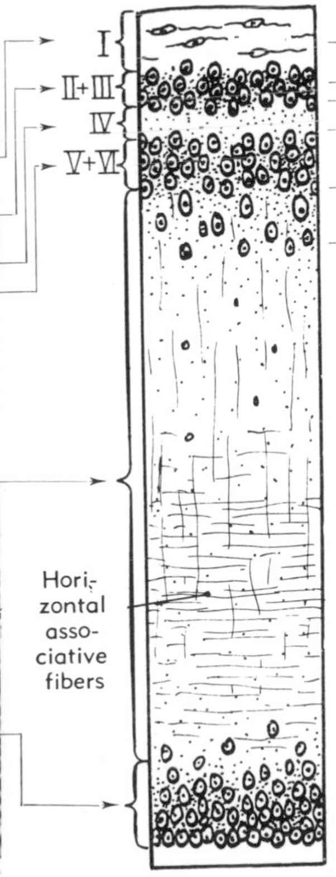

I
II + III
IV
V + VI

Horizontal associative fibers

Fig. 8. — About 100 days.

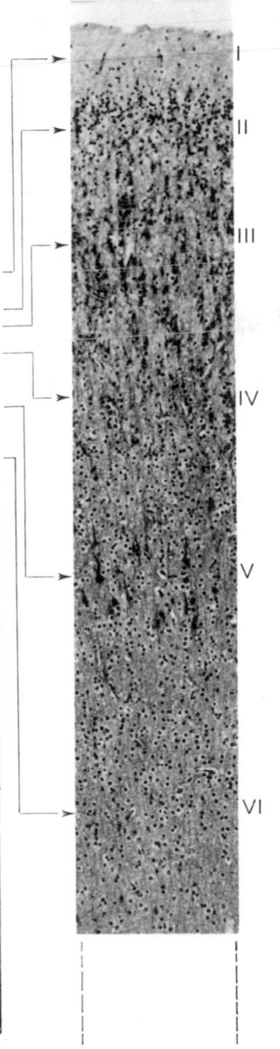

I
II
III
IV
V
VI

Fig. 9. — About 6 months (× 75).

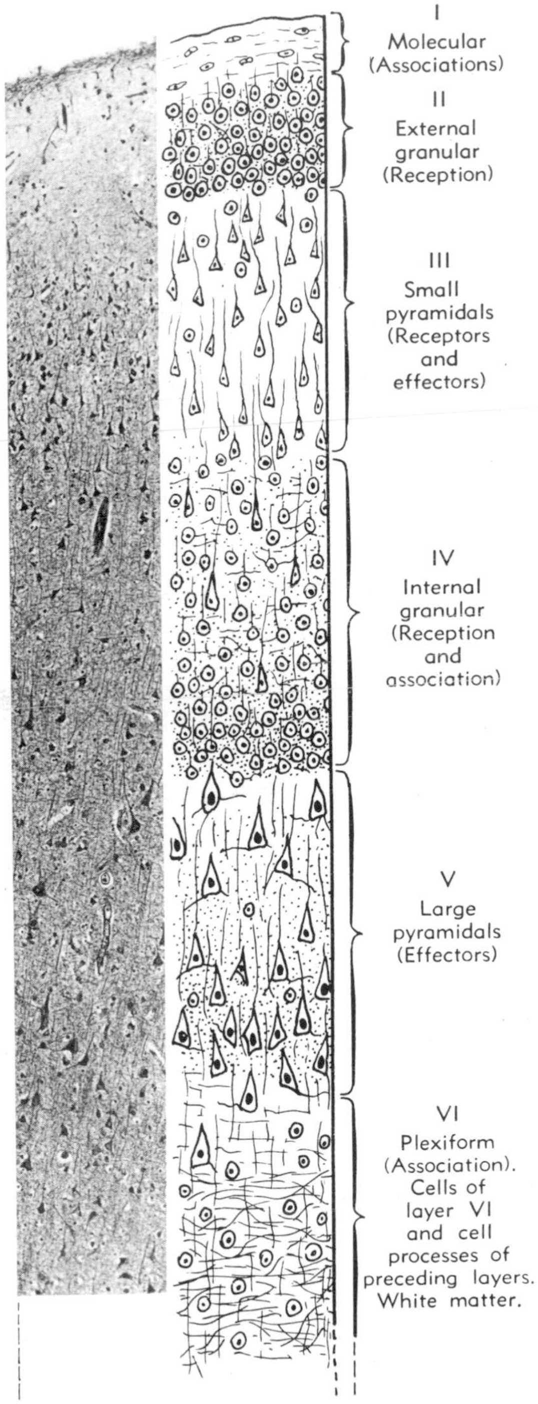

I Molecular (Associations)
II External granular (Reception)
III Small pyramidals (Receptors and effectors)
IV Internal granular (Reception and association)
V Large pyramidals (Effectors)
VI Plexiform (Association). Cells of layer VI and cell processes of preceding layers. White matter.

Fig. 10. — Adult (×75)(see also fig. 2, p. 80).

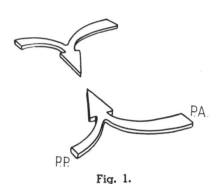

Fig. 1.

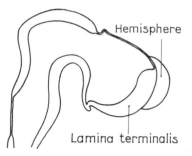

Fig. 1 a. — *Median sagittal section of a human fetus of about 36 days.*

The telecenphalic commissures are the fiber systems which connect homologous parts of the two cortical hemispheres. The fibers produced by the right and left cortex cross in the midline, forming the commissures. This takes place in the lamina terminalis. This is the zone of junction of the two telencephalic vesicles, corresponding to the closure of the anterior neuropore.

1. **The anterior white commissure** (shown in white in the figures) connects the two olfactory bulbs by its anterior processes (P.A., fig. 1) and the two convolutions of the hippocampus by its posterior processes (P.P., fig. 1). It appears toward the end of the 2nd month. Its fibers pass in the inferior portion of the lamina terminalis.

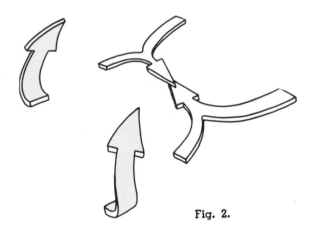

Fig. 2.

2. **The trigonum** (in yellow) connects the two hippocampi and the two palocortices by the hippocampal commissures (C.H., fig. 3). This appears during the 3rd month. Its fibers, coming from the posterior pillars of the fornix (Pi. P., fig. 4) pass in the middle portion of the lamina terminalis. It partially regresses after appearance of the corpus callosum [1].

The white commissure and trigonum belong to the rhinencephalon. They are found only in lower vertebrates.

3. **The corpus callosum** (in green) connects the two parts of the neocortex. Its primordia appear in the 3rd month. The commissure forms in the superior portion of the lamina terminalis. It develops in an anterior-posterior direction, parallel with the neocortex (*green arrow, fig. 5 a*), and

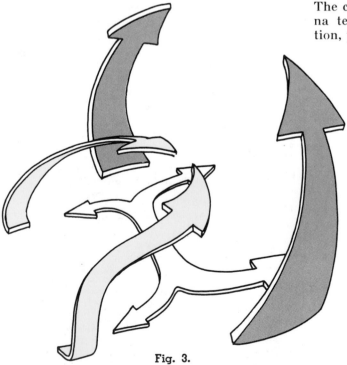

Fig. 3.

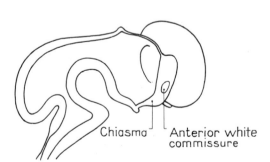

Chiasma   Anterior white commissure

Fig. 3 a. — *About 55 days.*

[1] The anterior pillars (Pi. A.) connect the mammillary tubercules. They form a diencephalic commissure. The anterior and posterior pillars of the same side join the hippocampus and the homolateral mammillary tubercle. They do not therefore form a commissure but a system of intrahemispheric association.

COMMISSURES

its sixe varies with that of the neocortex. In man, they are both large. The corpus callosum is not fully formed until the 6th month.

Between the corpus callosum and the subjacent trigonum, there is a loss of material forming the narrow cavity of the septum lucidum (fig. 3, p. 67).

It may be noted that the rhinencephalic commissures appear before the neocortical commissure. This results from the progressive maturation of the various cortices and corresponds to the phylogenetic order.

Functional unity of the two hemispheres and, more generally, of the two halves of the symmetrical CNS is assured by the systems of association. There are, in fact, commissures in the subjacent layers and even in the cord.

Pathology. — The most frequently affected development is that of the corpus callosum. This may involve total or partial agenesis, or hypogenesis, with an abnormally thin corpus callosum. Morphogenesis of this commissure shows that there are at least two possible causes of derangement:

— a deficiency of the neocortical regions producing fibers;

— a deficiency of the pathway, the lamina terminalis.

Callosal agenesis (about 2 % of cases of cephalic pathology) most often results in debility and epilepsy [1]. Some cases are of genetic origin.

Since differentiation of the corpus callosum is very prolonged, clinical procedures such as use of X-rays may be dangerous even if they are used late in pregnancy.

[1] For some types there are no clinical examples. The callosal fibers reach the neocortex via the anterior white commissure. This corresponds to the reappearance in man of a system normally found in lower mammals without a callosal commissure.

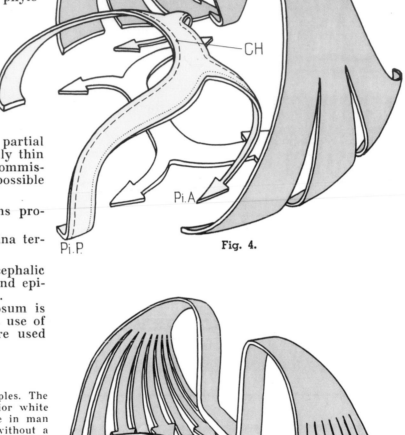

Fig. 4.

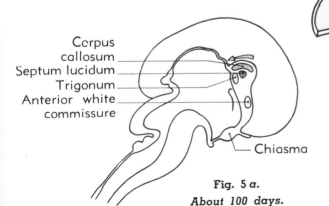

Corpus callosum
Septum lucidum
Trigonum
Anterior white commissure
Chiasma

Fig. 5 a.
About 100 days.

Fig. 5.

MENINGES

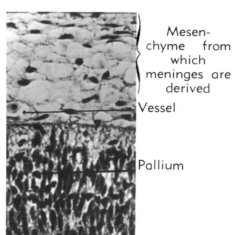

Mesen-
chyme from
which
meninges are
derived

Vessel

Pallium

Fig. 1. — *Human embryo of about 40 days* (× 425).

The meninges are membranes which are interposed between the bone (cranial vault or spine) and the central nervous system. They completely enclose the central nervous system. They consist of:

— **the soft or leptomeninges,** the pia mater and the arachnoid. They are derived from ectomesenchyme from the neural crests, according to evidence from ablation and grafting experiments in amphibians and birds as well as histological and histochemical evidence in mammals. The pia mater lies directly on the nervous tissue. The arachnoid surrounds the blood vessels (fig. 3);

— **the hard meninges or dura mater,** which is derived from ordinary mesenchyme and differentiates after the leptomeninges. Normal development of the meninges is dependant on that of the CNS.

Role of the meninges. — *Protection against mechanical shock.*

— *Vascular role.* The pia mater and the arachnoid accompany the vessels penetrating the nervous tissue (fig. 3). This sheathing takes place at the level of the capillaries which are then directly in contact with the neuroglial cells (1).

— *Emunctory role.* Resorption of the cerebrospinal fluid takes place in the subarachnoid spaces.

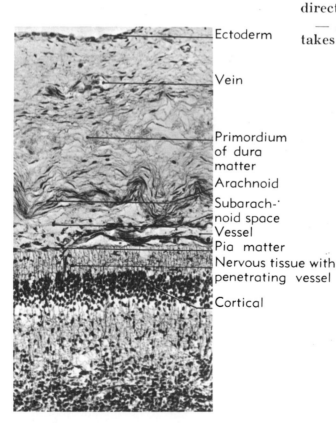

Ectoderm

Vein

Primordium
of dura
matter

Arachnoid

Subarach-
noid space

Vessel

Pia matter

Nervous tissue with
penetrating vessel

Cortical

Fig. 2. — *Human embryo of about 65 days* (× 170).

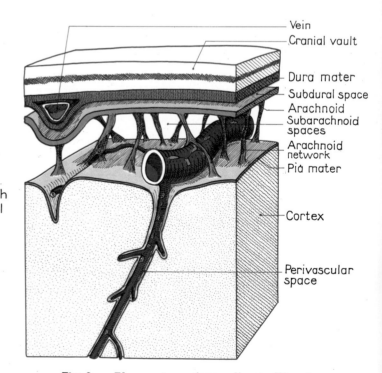

Vein

Cranial vault

Dura mater

Subdural space

Arachnoid

Subarachnoid
spaces

Arachnoid
network

Pia mater

Cortex

Perivascular
space

Fig. 3. — *The meninges* (according to WEED).

(1) The combination formed by the capillary wall and the neuroglial cells comprises the blood-brain barrier, impermeable to some microbes and some compounds (antibiotics), permeable to others (sulfonamides). This barrier is formed slowly, and is not present in the young embryo.

CHOROID PLEXES

THE CHOROID PLEXES

In the regions where the ependymal wall is thin (roofs of the 3rd and 4th ventricles and internal portion of lateral ventricles) the leptomeninges push this wall into the ventricles, forming the primordia of the choroid plexes (fig. 4, 5, and 6). The plexes thus form a richly vascularized meningeal axis covered with thin cuboidal ependymal epithelium, apparently secretory.

The first choroid plexes develop in the 4th ventricle between the 48th and the 50th day (embryo about 20 mm).

Role of the plexes. — *Production of cerebrospinal fluid.* The cerebrospinal fluid circulates toward the 4th ventricle and the spinal canal. It then passes through the foramina of Magendie and Luschka and is resorbed in the subarachnoid spaces (arrows, fig. 6). In the fetus, cerebrospinal fluid may furnish proteins to the CNS during its development.

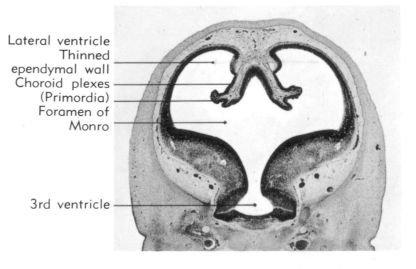

Lateral ventricle
Thinned ependymal wall
Choroid plexes (Primordia)
Foramen of Monro

3rd ventricle

Fig. 4. — *Human fetus, about 50 days.*
Frontal section (× 15).

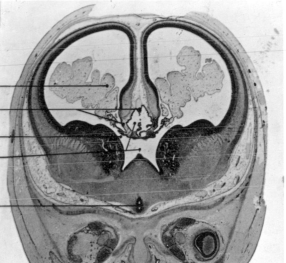

Choroid plexes
Thinned ependymal wall
Foramen of Monro
3rd ventricle

3rd ventricle

Fig. 5. — *Human fetus, about 65 days.*
Frontal section (× 6).

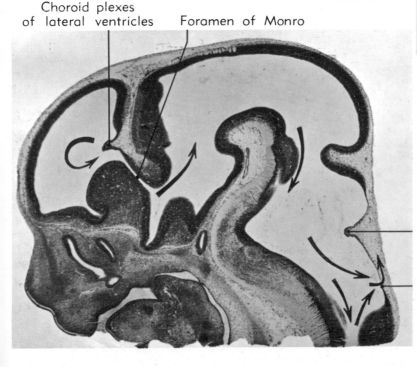

Choroid plexes of lateral ventricles   Foramen of Monro

Choroid plexes of 4th ventricle

Foramen of Luschka

Fig. 6. — *Rat fetus of 15 days.*
Paramedian sagittal section (× 20).

VASCULARIZATION

Cephalic circulation begins to be established very early, at the 7-somite stage (3 weeks), while the neural groove is not yet closed (fig. 1). It develops very rapidly, along with the encephalon.

The prosencephalon is irrigated first, by the internal carotids, the extremities of the dorsal aortas. Vascularization of the rhombencephalon and of the mesencephalon occurs later. These networks are derived from the basilar artery, which is formed from the confluence of the vertebral arteries.

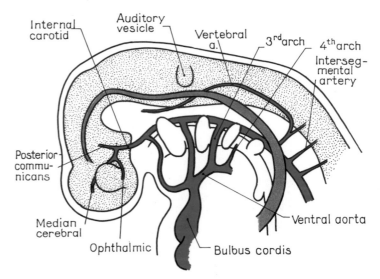

Fig. 1. — *Human fetus of about 21 days* (2 mm).

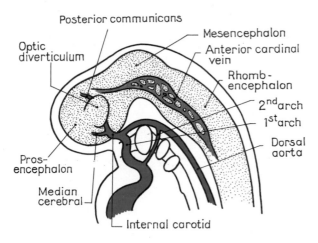

Fig. 2. — *Human fetus of about 24 days* (3 mm).

Fig. 3. — *Human fetus of about 26 days* (4 mm).

These arteries join together to form Willis's circle, definitively formed by 7 1/2 to 8 weeks (shown in dark red in figures 4, 6, and 8). With its own regulatory system to project it from too wide fluctuations, this network provides the encephalon with the large quantity of blood it needs: 15 % of the total amount.

Willis's circle is nourished by blood richer in oxygen than that of the other parts of the body. In fact, most of the oxygenated blood coming from the placenta bypasses the right ventricle by the foramen of Botal (foramen ovale) and passes directly into the left ventricle. Thus it does not mix with the venous blood of the circulation returning from the brain (superior vena cava), and leaves the heart by the aorta to pass first into the primitive carotids (fig. 7).

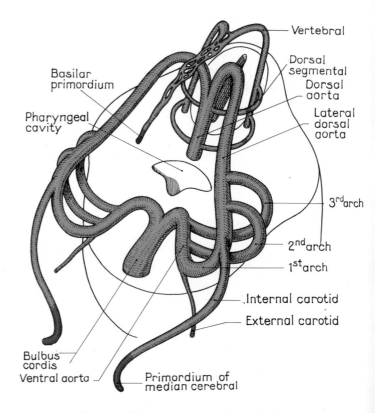

Fig. 4. — *Human fetus of about 26 days.*

OF ENCEPHALON

In contrast, the small portion of oxygenated blood which does not pass through the foramen ovale is caught in the venous current of the superior vena cava and passes into the right ventricle. It mixes with the venous blood and thus loses oxygen. The mixed blood then passes into the pulmonary artery, then the ductus arteriosus which reaches the aorta downstream from the primitive carotids (fig. 7). It is then distributed to the trunk and caudal parts of the embryo.

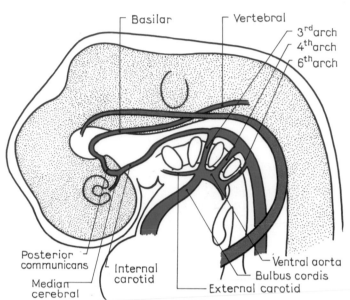

Fig. 5. — *Human fetus of about 31 days* (6 mm).

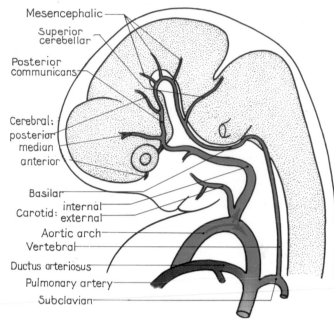

Fig. 7. — *Human fetus of about 50 days* (20 mm) (the venous return is not shown in this figure).

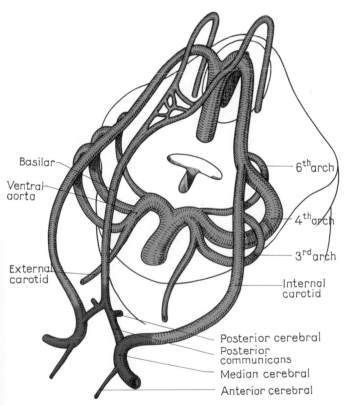

Fig. 6. — *Human fetus of about 31 days.*

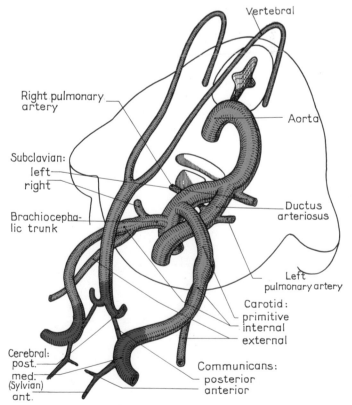

Fig. 8. — *Human fetus of about 50 days.*

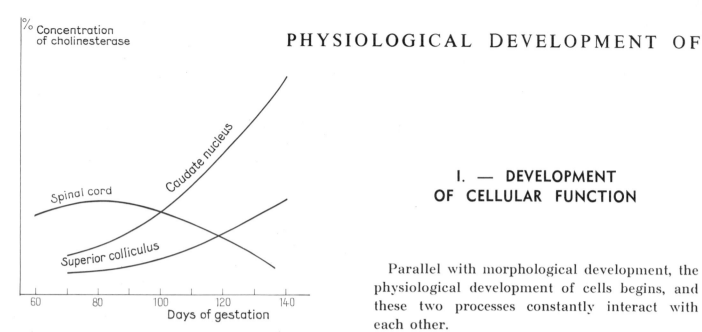

Fig. 1. — *Concentration of cholinesterase in spinal cord and brain in the sheep fetus* (according to NACHMANSOHN). Appearance of this enzyme characterizes beginning of maturation of the various systems. Its level serves as a measure of their activity.

I. — DEVELOPMENT OF CELLULAR FUNCTION

Parallel with morphological development, the physiological development of cells begins, and these two processes constantly interact with each other.

Characteristic enzyme systems appear first in spinal cord cells, then in those of the brain: succinic dehydrogenase, ATPase, phosphogluconate dehydrogenase, carbonic anhydrase, cytochrome oxidase, cholinesterase, etc. (fig. 1). Their levels increase greatly just after birth.

Appearance of the Nissl bodies (cytoplasmic RNA) marks the beginning of increased protein synthesis resulting in formation of axon processes and dendrites (fig. 2, and fig. 1, p. 10).

Signs of functional activity are superimposed on these morphological and chemical changes: the beginning of electrical activity, and reactivity resulting in muscular contractions, as well as suppression of the related reflexes by cephalic structures.

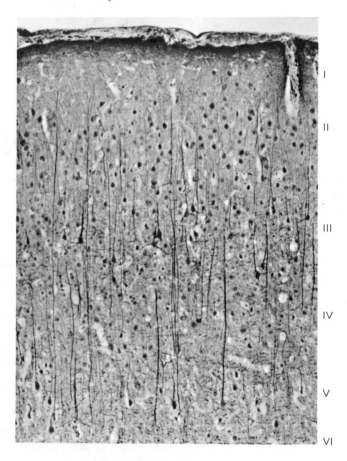

Fig. 2. — *Cortex of adult rat* ($\times$ 135). Note the dendritic processes going toward the cortical surface (silver impregnation). The cortical layers are numbered (see p. 73).

THE CENTRAL NERVOUS SYSTEM

II. — CEREBRAL MATURATION

Cerebral maturation is slower and more gradual than that of the rest of the CNS, and corresponds to the duration of cortical histogenesis. Physiologically, maturation may be evaluated by the spontaneous electrical activity of the brain recorded from the skull.

Electrical potentials recorded across the amniotic membrane suggest that this activity begins about the 50th day of intrauterine life. Its maturation, a function of dendritic development of the neurons and enzymatic development, is completed at about 14 years of age.

Fetus of about 7 months. — Anarchic activity with interhemispheric asymmetry (immature cortex and commissures).

Right hemisphere

Left hemisphere

1 second   *Fetus.*

At birth. — Slow, more coordinated activity (3-4 cycles/second), with beginning of symmetrization.

Birth.

From 2 to 3 years. — More rapid (alpha = 6 to 7 cycles/second), symmetrical, activity of greater amplitude, well organized in the occipital regions, less well in the frontal regions. Cerebral electrical maturation progresses in the posterior-anterior direction.

3 years.

In the adult (from 13-14 years). — Still more rapid activity (8-12 cycles/second). The alpha is well organized on the entire cerebral surface.

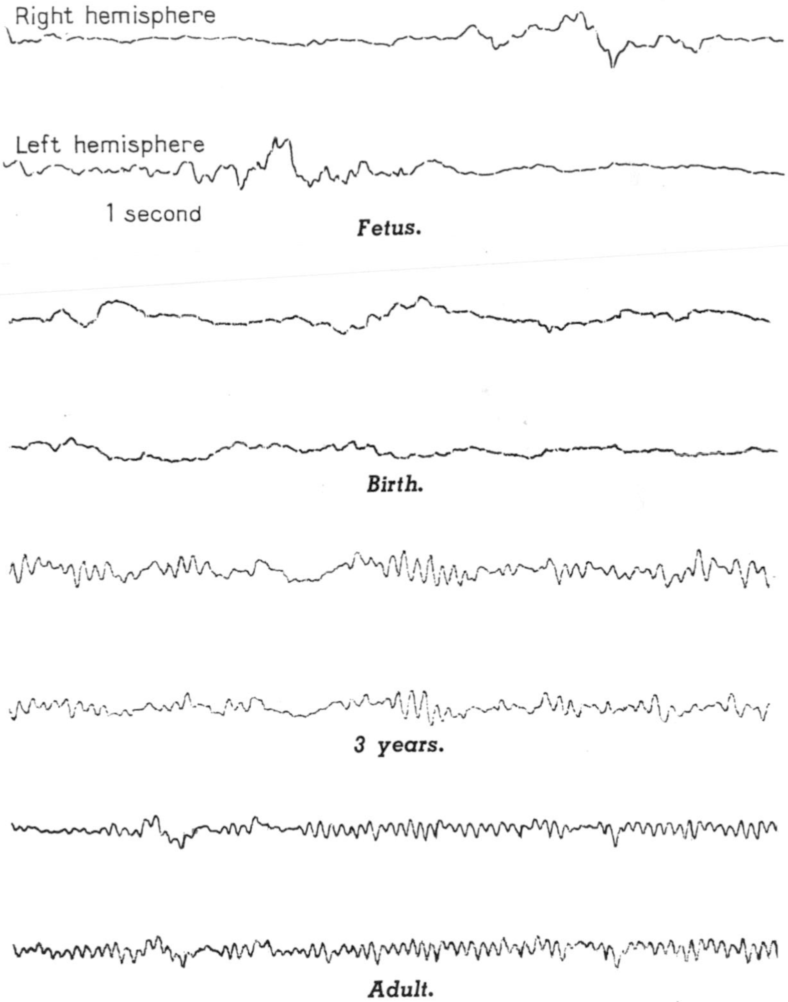

Adult.

Fig. 3.

During maturation of the brain there are special requirements for glycogen and especially oxygen. Although in the adult the oxygen consumption of the brain is 25% of that utilized by the entire body, in the newborn and the young child it may be as high as 60%. Neonatal anoxia is thus very serious and may cause intracranial hemorrhage, epilepsy, or psychomotor retardation.

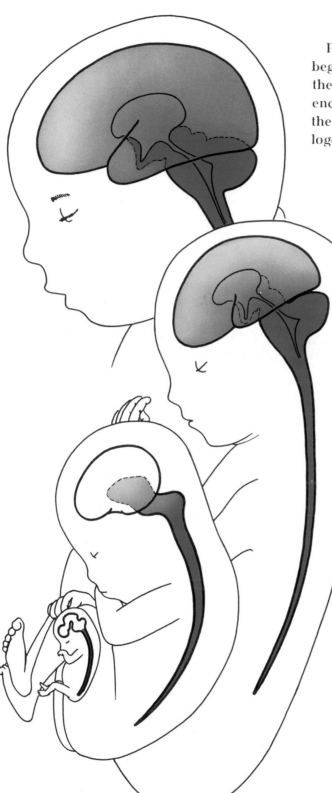

Fig. 1. — *Maturation of central nervous system.* Increasing intensity of the red color indicates the different degrees of maturation at 2, 4, 6, and 8 months.

Parallel with histogenesis, physiological development begins in the spinal cord, follows in the derivatives of the rhombencephalon, the mesencephalon, and the prosencephalon, and ends with the later development of the cerebral cortex. This progression conforms to phylogenetic evolution (fig. 1).

I. — FETAL STAGES

— First muscular reactions to external stimuli: 8th week.

— Spontaneous movements, sign of medullary maturation: 9th week.

— Osteotendinous reflexes: 6th month.

Respiratory center of the medulla is functional at 5 1/2 months. Since maturation of the pulmonary alveolar epithelium occurs at about 6 months of gestation, viability is theoretically possible at this age (see Volume II).

— Archaic reflexes (subcortical centers):

— sucking (5 months of gestation);

— grasping (6 months of gestation).

The inexcitability of the cerebral cortex until this time shows that these movements are independent of the cortex. They indicate only very rudimentary instinctive reactions like sucking and grasping, which are also seen in anencephalics.

— Cerebral maturation begins between 6 and 7 months, when the basic structures are completed. Some diseases, like diabetes, may slow down this development; such newborn infants have a psychomotor retardation of one or several months.

II. — POSTNATAL STAGES

The immediate postnatal period is, in terms of nervous function, a continuation of the fetal state. Behavior is reflex and purely subcortical. Movement is instinctual and rudimentary and consists only of flexion and extension or of reflexes such as crying and coughing.

DEVELOPMENT

The neocortex becomes excitable about the 10th day, but only in a weak and diffuse way. For a long time, movement is still awkward and generalized. Gradually, automatic movements come under cortical control and become more elaborate. Behavior becomes progressively imitative and expressive.

One of the structural developments which condition this progression may be followed in the cortex. The first fibers to be myelinated are those coming from the motor, visual, and auditory zones found in all mammals. The last, myelinated at the end of gestation and shortly after birth, are those coming from the association areas whose large size characterizes the human brain (fig. 2 and 3).

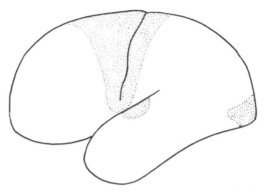

Fig. 2. — *The motor and sensory cortical surfaces in man. In white,* association areas.

Principal clinical stages. — Regression of archaic reflexes between 1 and 3 months.

— Complete and stable head-righting when lying prone at 3 months.

— Sitting at 8 or 9 months.

— Standing at 9 1/2 to 10 months.

— Walking at 12 to 15 months.

— First word between 18 months and 2 years.

— Cerebral maturation ends at about 14 years.

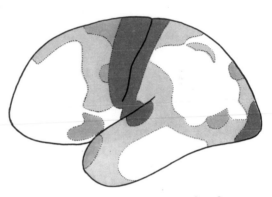

Fig. 3. — *Myelogenesis in the human brain* (modified from FLECHSIG). *Dark green :* areas where myelogenesis begins. *Medium green, light green, and white areas :* 2nd, 3rd, and 4th stages respectively of myelogenesis.

Overall development of the brain. — The cortex has a surface of about 700 cm² at birth, 950 cm² at 5 months, and 1,670 cm² at 2 years, after which the surface no longer increases.

At birth, the brain weighs from 300 to 340 g (1/10 of the body weight). Its weight and its volume increase most during the first two years of life. This growth occurs essentially in the hemispheres, in particular in the frontal lobes. The softness of the cranial sutures and the fontanelles permits this expansion. Increase of brain weight continues until about 14 years of age, but more and more slowly. It is due especially to multiplication of neuroglial cells and to neuronal fibrillar growth, for the central nervous system has most of its neurons at the time of birth.

In the adult, the brain represents only about 2.5% of the body weight, since the total body mass grows considerably.

GENERAL ASPECTS

Brain malformations occur in about 0.54% of live births and in 2.97% of stillbirths. In girls, malformations of the nervous system are more numerous than cardiac or digestive system malformations. In boys, the incidence of nervous system malformations falls between those of the other two systems.

As in all other organs, brain malformations may be caused in three ways:

— *exogenous causes:* nutritional, physical (x-rays especially), viral, parasitic, and chemical. Medications are an important part of the last group;

— *endogenous causes,* hereditary, poorly defined except in some cases (Tay-Sachs disease, trisomy 13-15);

— *interaction of exogenous and endogenous factors.* Differences in sensitivity to exogenous factors occur according to species and strain. So far such interactions have been demonstrated only in experimental animals.

Teratogenic factors can act for a long time since brain development takes place over an extended period. Theoretically, problems affecting general development can be distinguished from those affecting histogenesis, but actually the two are most often related.

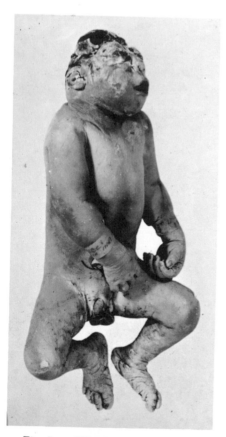

Fig. 1. — *Human anencephalic at term.*

PROBLEMS OF NEURAL GROOVE CLOSURE

1. Anencephalus

Anencephalus results from an arrest of neural groove closure in the brain. It is thus a disorder of early embryogenesis. It is caused by defective induction of the prechordal plate or the parachordal mesoderm, or poor receptivity of the competent neural plate.

The overall structure of the brain is disturbed. The hemispheres develop below the region of telencephalic evagination (fig. 2) and the edges of the diencephalic groove cover them (fig. 3).

MALFORMATIONS

As in typical spina bifida, the nervous tissue is not covered with bone or skin. The cranial vault, like the posterior arch of the vertebrae, differentiates only under the influence of a normal neural tube. The skin is in continuity with the nervous tissue, as in the neural groove stage.

However, normal histogenesis occurs until the beginning of neocortical differentiation. But several weeks before term, vascular problems lead to general necrosis so that only choroid plexes, some nerves, and degenerating nervous tissue persist.

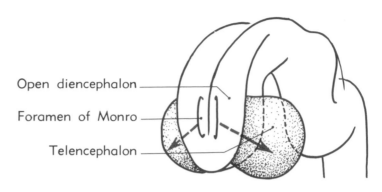

Open diencephalon

Foramen of Monro

Telencephalon

Fig. 2.

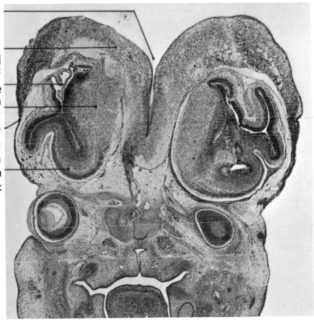

3rd ventricle

Diencephalon
Choroid
plexus of
lateral ventricle
Telencephalon
Junction of
neural tissue
and surface
ectoderm
Primordium
of cortex

Fig. 3. — *Anencephalus in a rat fetus of 17 days* (hypervitaminosis A in the mother, according to GIROUD). Frontal section at level of the eyes.

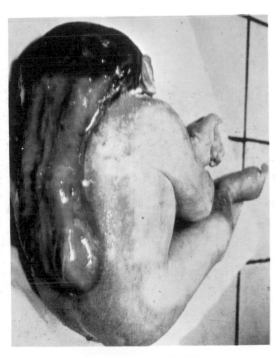

Fig. 4. — *Craniorachischisis.*

Anencephalus results in neonatal death in several minutes or several days.

A particularly extreme form of this anomaly is craniorachischisis, where the neural groove remains open throughout its length (fig. 4).

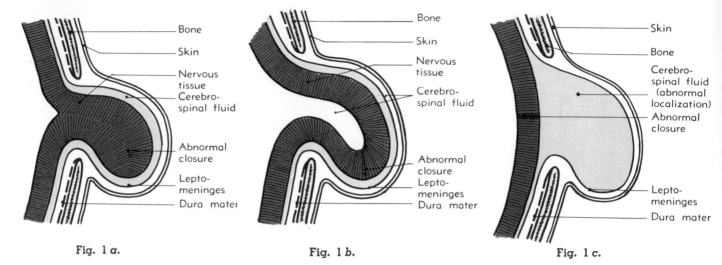

Fig. 1 a. Fig. 1 b. Fig. 1 c.

2. *Encephalocele and meningocele*

In addition to anencephalus, there are other more localized defects connected with closure of the encephalic neural groove.

— **Encephalocele** is the most serious type, most often untreatable. Part of the brain is herniated under the skin through a hole in the skull (fig. 1*a* and *b,* and fig. 2, 3, and 4).

— **Meningocele,** hernia of the meninges is compatible with life and can be treated surgically (fig. 1*c*).

These anomalies usually occur on the midline because of their origin.

The localized nature of the defect of groove closure explains why bone can form normally in the lateral portions. Similarly, the small extent of the opening allows the nervous tissue and skin at the edges to join more or less well at a later stage. Nevertheless, the skin is always abnormal, fine, parchment-like and hairless. These characteristics are like those of the minor forms of spina bifida. In certain cases, however, the abnormality of closure is evident (fig. 4).

Experimentally, many agents may be used to produce these malformations; X-rays, anoxia, nutritional deficiencies, hypervitaminosis A, tissue antibodies, and certain drugs.

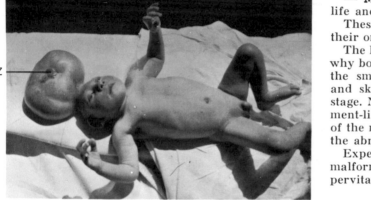

Fig. 2. — *Enormous encephalocele in a fetus at term.* Z : ulcerated zone corresponding to a localized failure of neural groove closure. Survival : 74 days. Normal archaic reflexes.

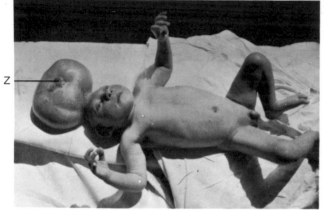

Fig. 3. — *Neural axis of the newborn shown in figure 2.* Anterior view.

1 : ulcerated zone removed.
2 : extracranial portion of hemispheres distended with cerebrospinal fluid.
3 : intracranial portion of hemispheres.
4 : cerebellum.
5 : medulla.
6 : spinal cord with cauda equina at right.

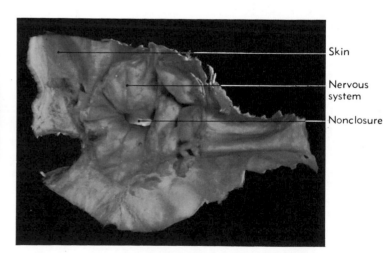

Fig. 4. — *The removed ulcerated zone, internal view.* The junction of skin and nervous tissue looks like a buttonhole.

CYCLOCEPHALUS

Cyclocephalus is a rather rare malformation involving only the prosencephalic derivatives. The telencephalon does not subdivide into two hemispheres and its single cavity communicates with the 3rd ventricle by a single duct (fig. 6). Since the neural groove is closed, the cranial vault and skin are normal. There is only one median eye (cyclopia) or considerable hypertelorism. Usually there is no hypophysis. The nasal apparatus is more or less atrophied and is often replaced by a trunk, with a single median orifice instead of two nasal orifices.

This malformation is due to defective induction of the prechordal plate, as has been shown experimentally. Excision of the prechordal plate brings about a concentration of cerebral elements on the midline and secondarily cyclopia.

Among the teratogenic agents used experimentally, hypervitaminosis A and X-rays can produce this malformation. The fetus shows either the severe type or the minor types, with the hemispheres separate and nearly normal dorsally. In man, a chromosome defect is now suspected as the possible cause of this anomaly.

Cyclocephalus causes death. However, some children with a minor type of the malformation have been known to live for several years.

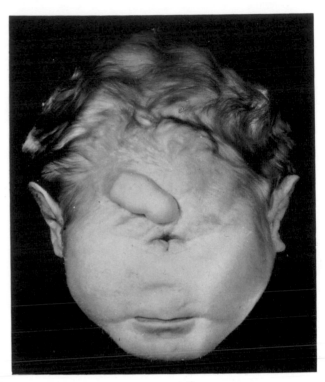

Fig. 5. — *Cyclocephalus at term.*

ARHINENCEPHALUS

Arhinencephalus is probably in the general category of cyclocephalus. In addition to the dysgenesis of the rhinencephalon which characterizes it, there is general atrophy of the telencephalon which remains more or less univesicular. There are also malformations of the intermaxillary segment whose development is related to that of the rhinencephalon: cleft lip, agenesis of the nasal septum with median union of the nostrils, a single nasal fossa, and hypotelorism.

Absence or hypogenesis of the rhinencephalon is due to a disorder of the olfactory placodes which do not produce fibers and therefore do not induce formation of the olfactory bulbs. The initial cause of this problem, as in cyclocephalus, might be defective induction by the prechordal plate. Some cases are genetic (trisomy 13-15).

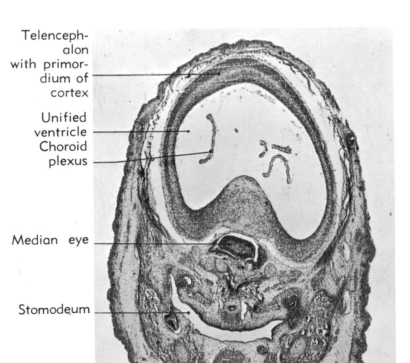

Telencephalon with primordium of cortex

Unified ventricle Choroid plexus

Median eye

Stomodeum

Fig. 6. — *Frontal section of a cyclocephalic mouse fetus of 18 days, produced by hypervitaminosis A in the mother.* (According to GIROUD, DELMAS, and MARTINET.)

Normal sutures

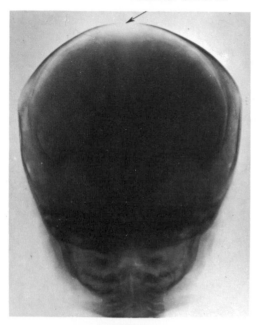

Fig. 1. — *Radiograph of skull of a normal newborn.*

Disjunction of sutures

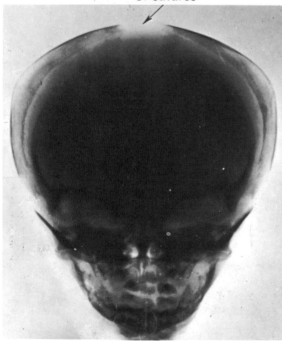

Fig. 2. — *Radiograph of skull of hydrocephalic newborn.*

Hydrocephalus is a frequent anomaly compatible with life. It is characterized by abnormal accumulation of cerebrospinal fluid in the ventricles or, in case of external hydrocephalus, in the subarachnoid spaces.

The mode of production of the cerebrospinal fluid, its circulation and resorption (see p. 77) indicate the three possible causes of hydrocephalus:

— excess production (communicating hydrocephalus);

— obstruction of circulation (noncommunicating hydrocephalus);

— defective resorption (communicating hydrocephalus).

In the majority of cases, hydrocephalus in the newborn is thought to be caused by an obstruction in the aqueduct of Sylvius, due to an anomaly, inflammation, or tumor.

Some types of hydrocephalus are due to obliteration of the orifices of the 4th ventricle. In some cases of spina bifida, in fact, the posterior portion of the brain is sunk in the occipital opening. This is the Arnold-Chiari syndrome. With caudal elongation of the trunk, the spinal cord, which is stuck to the skin because of the spina bifida, follows the movement and pulls the brain posteriorly.

In several cases there is a recessive, sex-linked genetic anomaly, transmitted by the X chromosome. Hydrocephalus does not appear in the females who transmit it, but is manifested in 50% of the males. In these cases, there is usually overproduction of cerebrospinal fluid.

Hydrocephalus causes increased size of the head (normally 35 to 40 cm circumference), an enlargement of the cranial sutures (fig. 1 and 2), progressive thinning of the bone of the cranium, and when it is very severe, lamination of the cerebral cortex. Usually it is accompanied by psychological retardation which may be severe enough to cause debility, convulsions, or cerebral motor disability. There is now surgical treatment which can stabilize the condition of the patient by removing the obstruction. This treatment is, however, without effect on the nervous lesions already produced.

MICROCEPHALUS

In microcephalus there is a small brain inside a small cranium.

Some cases are genetic. Others may be due to pelvic X-ray during pregnancy, or to toxoplasmosis.

Developmental arrest occurs at late stages of gestation. Problems of cellular multiplication or migration may be involved. Cellular densities may be abnormally low or the cortical layers may be less numerous than normally. Microcephalus is accompanied by mental deficiency and sometimes convulsions.

DYSGENESIS

Anomalies of dysgenesis involve agenesis or degeneration of certain cellular groups.

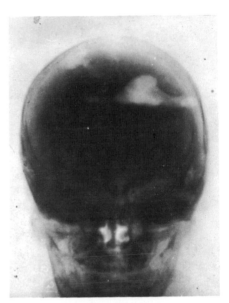

Fig. 3. — *Porencephalus.*

— In *porencephalus*, for example, a lateral ventricle communicates with the corresponding subarachnoid spaces by an opening (fig. 3). It is thought that these anomalies are due to a defect of vascularization. They often result in debility, convulsions, and cerebral motor disability.

— *Agenesis of corpus callosum:* see p. 75.

— *Hemispheric or cerebellar agenesis or hypogenesis,* similarly due to early vascular problems, is seen rather rarely.

HETEROTOPY

Rosettes. — Rosettes are small accessory paraependymal cavities, and may or may not be connected to the principal cavity. They are surrounded by a germinal layer which can give rise to nervous cells. The disorders produced by rosettes vary according to their localization. They have been produced experimentally by vitamin deficiency or X-rays.

Congenital myxedema. — Thyroid deficiency brings about defective cellular migration at certain points. Differentiation then occurs at the original site, causing heterotopies which cause problems.

ANOMALIES OF THE CORTICAL SURFACES

Anomalies of the cortical surfaces include lissencephaly (absence of convolutions), micro- or pachygyry (too small or too large convolutions), most often associated with other cerebral malformations. They are always accompanied by debility or idiocy. Their pathogenesis is unknown.

SENSE ORGANS

NEUROSENSORY

Neurosensory integration is achieved through permanent interactions between the sense organs and the central nervous system. These interactions permit the individual to adapt to a given situation.

In vertebrates the CNS and the exteroceptive sense organs are derived from the ectoderm. As suggested by this common origin, their relationship is very close and is clearly apparent during evolution. Study of anatomy and comparative embryology shows that the sensory and nervous cells differentiate progressively from a single cellular category, the neurosensory cells, which are also derived from ectoderm.

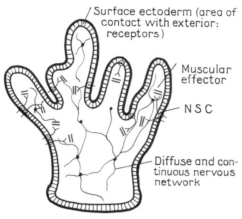

Fig. 1. — *Coelenterates.*

Surface ectoderm (area of contact with exterior: receptors)

Muscular effector

N S C

Diffuse and continuous nervous network

Differentiation of these cells allows:

— grouping of homologous cells, sensory or nervous;

— connections between nervous structures, which increase in number as these structures become more abundant.

These two processes determine neurosensory integration.

COELENTERATES

In coelenterates, the receptors are isolated and diffuse cells, the neurosensory cells (NSC). Their essential characteristic is sensitivity to both exciting and conducting inputs. In addition, they react to diverse excitations; they are not specialized.

The rudimentary structure of such a system explains why the animal is more capable of reactions than of adaptation.

WORMS

In the more evolved invertebrates like the worms, there are basic advances as compared with coelenterates (fig. 2).

a) The primordia of some neurosensory cells (NSC) are grouped, expecially in the head, and form a thick area of surface ectoderm, the placode. The NSC which are derived from this are therefore grouped into a localized sensory organ (LSO), more or less specialized.

b) Other NSC migrate deeply and give rise to motor neurons (M): neurosensory cells and purely nervous cells are distinct.

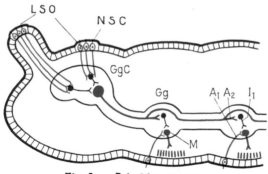

LSO
NSC
GgC
Gg
A_1 A_2 I_1
M

Fig. 2. — *Primitive worms.*

c) Under the influence of NSC, several motor cells unite into ganglia (Gg): the nervous system becomes concentrated. In each ganglion interneurons appear permitting intraganglionic connections (I_1). The largest ganglion is that of the cephalic end (GgC); it corresponds to the placodal afferents. It sends connective fibers to the caudal end.

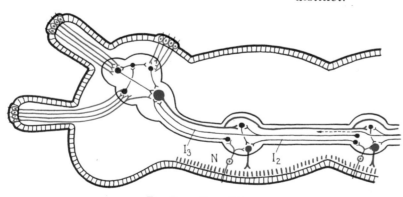

I_3
N
I_2

Fig. 3. — *Annelids.*

d) Diverse afferents thus come together in a ganglionic cell: A_1, metameric afferent; A_2, cephalic afferent. *The convergence of at least two afferents in the same*

INTEGRATION

effector cell is the simplest mechanism of neurosensory integration. This mechanism exists not only at the cellular level, but also at the level of general organization. Several systems of specialized information (eye, antenna) come together in the cephalic ganglia.

In the most evolved worms, the annelids (fig. 3), the number and size of placodes increases and the sensory organs derived from them are more complex and more specialized. Besides, the nuclei of certain NSC migrate deeply with part of the cytoplasm (N). This is the beginning of dissociation of receptors and conductors which is achieved in the vertebrates (fig. 5). Long, intermetameric neurons appear (I₂, I₃); they increase the possibility of connections. The cephalic ganglia thus receive more information. One part tends to govern the whole, unity begins, and behavior is more adaptive.

However, despite these advances, none of the different parts of the CNS of worms centralizes all information. Responses remain very segmental and adaptation is limited.

VERTEBRATES

The ganglionic system of invertebrates is replaced in vertebrates by the spinal cord and the brain. Nervous and sensory concentration becomes intense, especially cephalically (parallelism between cephalization of sens organs and that of the CNS, p. 13).

The sensory ganglia (G.S.) connected to the CNS contain numerous purely conductor cells. The receptor-conductor dissociation begun in the invertebrates is achieved. There are now sensory cells, conductor cells (sensory ganglionic cells and interneurons) and motor cells (fig. 5). With an increased number of neural elements, this last dissociation multiples the possibilities of connections. These are still increased by the immense number of interneurons, tens of billions in man, which are interposed between the sensory afferents and the motor effectors.

Thus in vertebrates, and especially in man, afference no longer stops at the metamere. All information converges toward the enormous associative centers of the brain. Neurosensory integration and the adaptation which results from it are maximal.

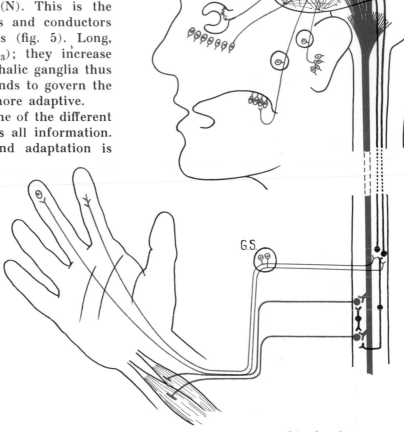

Fig. 4. — **Man.** The multitude of neurons of association in the brain are shown in black.

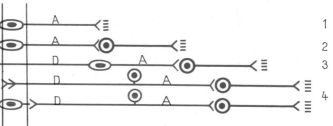

Fig. 5. — *Evolution of the receptor-effector system.* The interneurons are not shown.

A : axon. D : dendrite. The numbers correspond to the numbers of the preceding figures.

The placodes are localized thickenings of the cephalic surface ectoderm. Each placode is formed from a group of cells which gives rise to a specific organ with a given specialized function. The placodes include:

— the sensory placodes from which originate cephalic sense organs or some of their constituents;

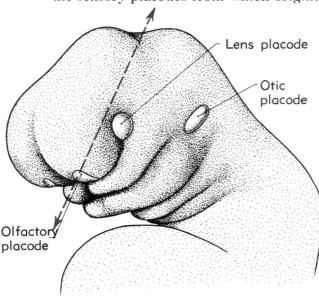

Fig. 1. — *Cephalic end of a human embryo of about 32 days, showing the placodes.*

— thickening of the stomodeal surface ectoderm from which the glandular hypophysis originates (see fig. 1, p. 20).
We will consider here only the sensory placodes.

In invertebrates, development of these placodes is simple. They are localized concentrations of surface ectodermal cells which give rise to neurosensory cells, specialized in the same function.

In vertebrates, development of these placodes is much more complex. At the end of neurulation, the surface ectoderm differentiates. However, in some areas of the cephalic extremity, the potentialities of the ectoderm are retained. Some very localized regions thicken according to a process analagous to that of the neural plate. These are the placodes (fig. 2).

Development of the placodes occurs at several times and in various ways:

— instead of remaining superficial, as in invertebrates, they penetrate the subjacent mesenchyme;

After this, they furnish not only neurosensory cells like those of the olfactory epithelium, but also distinct nervous and sensory cells, like those derived from the auditory vesicle. In the lens (optic) placode, differentiation is entirely different. The lens is neither sensory nor nervous;

— structures derived from the various placodes relate with specialized areas of the brain.

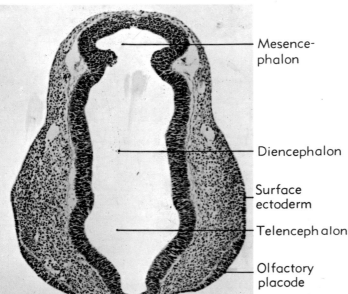

Fig. 2. — *Cephalic end of a human embryo of about 30 days* ($\times$ 65). The plane of section is shown by the arrow in figure 1.

PLACODES

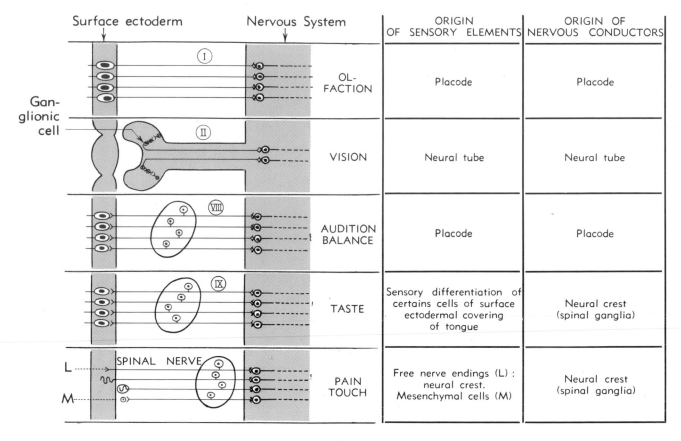

Fig. 3.

Figure 3 shows:

— that all sensory cells come from the surface ectoderm except those of touch and the eye. These latter are derived directly from the CNS. Their nature, concentration, and specialization are however analogous to those of the placodal cells;

— that the olfactory and visual cells are typically neurosensory. These are the only examples of neurosensory cells in vertebrates. The olfactory nerve (I) thus appears to be a grouping of neurosensory elements, and the optic nerve (II), situated between the ganglionic cells of the retina and the neurons of the CNS appears to be a grouping of interneurons. They are different in this way from other sensory nerves (VIII, IX and spinal nerves).

We will study only the three exteroceptive sensory organs whose development involves a placode: *the olfactory, auditory, and visual systems.*

OLFACTORY

The primordia of the olfactory system consist of two placodes on the right and left of the anteroinferior portions of the frontal prominence. They appear about the 30th day, that is, after the optic and otic placodes. At this time the neural tube is completely closed. They are induced first by the adjacent mesoderm and secondarily by the ventral face of the prosencephalon (fig. 2, p. 94).

Although they appear last, we shall study them first because of their relatively simple development.

Each placode invaginates in the direction of the suprajacent brain (fig. 2 and 3). The stratified placodal base of the invagination forms the olfactory epithelium. The lateral walls form the ordinary surface ectodermal covering of the nasal cavities (fig. 3).

The placodal cells differentiate into neurosensory cells within the thickness of the epithelium. At about 1½ months, the deep pole of the superficial cells gives rise to an axon which crosses the epithelium and the mesenchyme, and makes contact with the olfactory zones of the telencephalon (fig. 4 a). Arrival of these fibers at the telencephalon induces formation of the olfactory bulbs (fig. 4 b, c, d, and fig. 2, p. 71). The axons then connect with the specialized structures of the CNS corresponding to the olfactory sensory system: the bulbs (fig. 5) connected with the olfactory cortical areas (fig. 1 c, p. 70).

Towards the end of the 3rd month, the mesenchyme between the sensory epithelium and the bulb gives rise to a cartilaginous structure, the lamina cribosa of the ethnoid which is organized around networks of the olfactory nerve and dissociates them (fig. 4 d and 5).

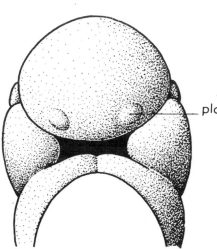

Fig. 1. — *Cephalic end of a human embryo of about 30 days.* Anterior view.

placode

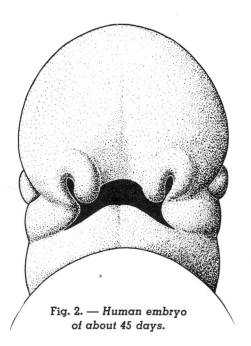

Fig. 2. — *Human embryo of about 45 days.*

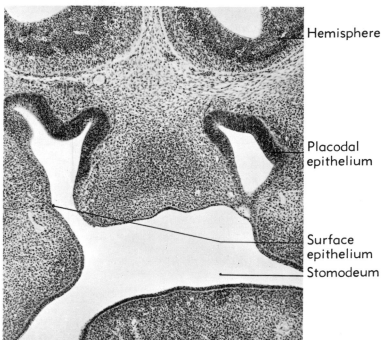

Hemisphere

Placodal epithelium

Surface epithelium

Stomodeum

Fig. 3. — *Frontal section of olfactory fossae of a rat embryo of 15 days* (× 30) (corresponds to a human embryo of about 45-50 days).

SYSTEM

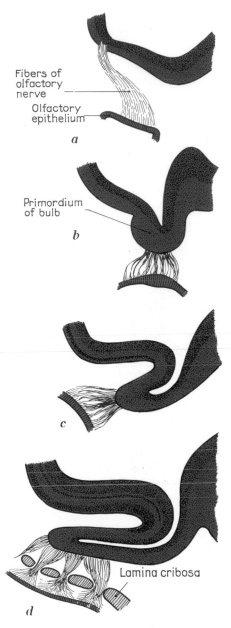

Fibers of olfactory nerve

Olfactory epithelium

a

Primordium of bulb

b

c

Lamina cribosa

d

Fig. 4. — *Human embryos.*

a) about 46 days (17 mm).
b) about 54 days (25 mm).
c) about 68 days (45 mm).
d) about 84 days (78 mm).

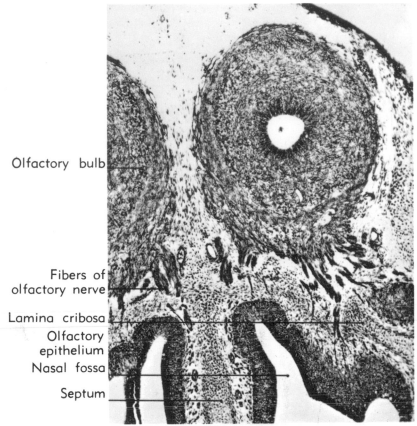

Olfactory bulb

Fibers of olfactory nerve

Lamina cribosa

Olfactory epithelium

Nasal fossa

Septum

Fig. 5. — *Newborn rat fetus.*
Frontal section ($\times$ 50).

MALFORMATIONS

Malformations of the olfactory organ are usually very serious, for they are always accompanied by anomalies of the CNS and the face. Because of this, they are in the category of more general malformations such as:

— **Cyclocephalus** (see p. 87). — In place of the nose, there is a proboscis with a single canal, resulting from the convergence of both nasal primordia on the midline. The sensory epithelium is very reduced or nonexistent. At the same time the olfactory bulbs may be absent. In some cases there may be two probosces or trunks. There are minor types of this malformation in which the nose is more or less cylindrical and the nasal fossae are closed.

Arhinencephalus (see p. 87).

In man, the causes of these malformations may be of genetic origin.

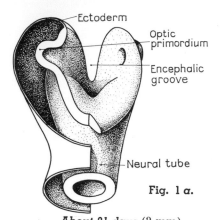

Fig. 1 a.

About 21 days (2 mm).
The embryo is viewed frontally.

Development of the eye involves two of the three germ layers: (1) the ectoderm, from which originate two elements of the visual system, the optic primordium and the lens primordium; and (2) the mesoderm, which furnishes the accessory structures.

The optic primordium appears very early. This is a lateral evagination which forms about the 18th day at the base of the future prosencephalon, before complete closure of the encephalic groove (fig. 1 a). It is induced by the prechordal plate. This evagination becomes a vesicle, the primary optic vesicle connected to the diencephalon by a peduncle (fig. 1 b and 2).

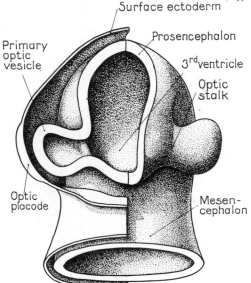

Fig. 1 b. — **About 27 days** (4 mm).

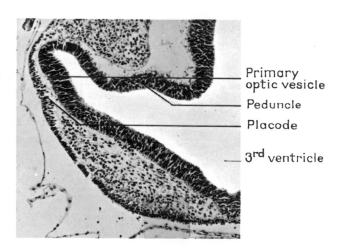

Fig. 2. — *Frontal section passing through optic primordium.* Human embryo of about 27 days (× 92).

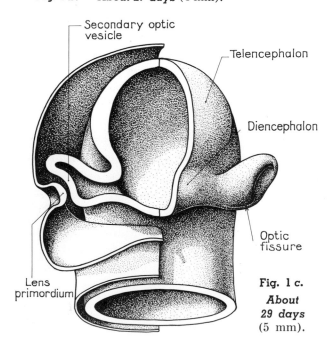

Fig. 1 c.
**About
29 days**
(5 mm).

The vesicle grows and invaginates, forming the secondary optic vesicle with two layers, internal and external (fig. 3, 4, and 5). Between the two layers, the intraretinal space communicates with the 3rd ventricle by the optic stalk. This space, almost non-existant in the adult, explains the possibility of detachment of the retina (fig. 3 and 4).

SYSTEM

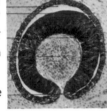

Intraretinal space
External layer
Internal layer
Lens primordium

Optic fissure

*Cross section along A-B
of figure 3.*
Rat fetus of 13 days (× 160).

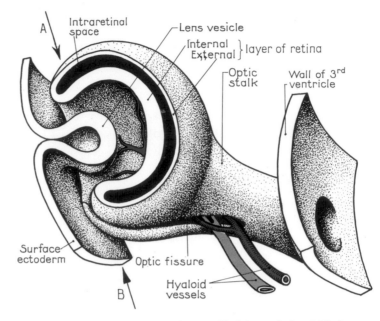

Fig. 3. — *Human ocular primordium.* Embryo of about 33 days.

Invagination of the vesicle also affects the optic stalk, forming the optic fissure. The hyaloid artery, the future central artery of the retina, penetrates the optic stalk through this fissure (fig. 3).

The lens primordium, or optic placode, results from a thickening of the cephalic surface ectoderm opposite to, and induced by, the optic vesicle (fig. 1 *b* and 2). This plate is rapidly depressed, giving a vesicle which is isolated from the surface ectoderm and bordered by only a single layer of cells. About the 40th day, the internal cells of the vesicle multiply and send out fibers towards the external cells (fig. 4). The earliest, central fibers form the nucleus of the lens (fig. 5). They soon become transparent because of the appearance of specific proteins. Growth of the lens by addition of new fibers at the periphery of the lens nucleus continues until the age of 20.

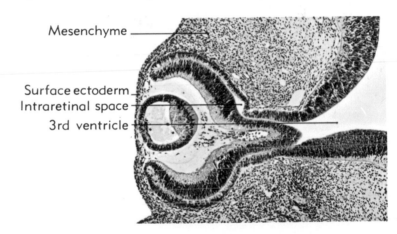

Fig. 4. — *Eye of human embryo of about 40 days* (× 100).

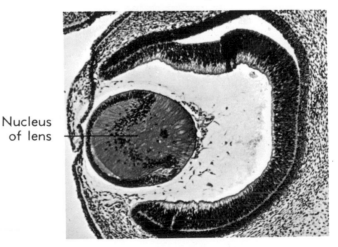

Fig. 5. — *Eye of human embryo of about 48 days* (× 120). The optic stalk is not seen in this figure.

1. *Differentiation of the secondary optic vesicle*: Pigment layer and neural layer of the retina. — The retina forms the body of the vesicle. The external layer remains simple and becomes the pigmented layer when small pigment granules appear in the epithelial cells. The internal layer provides the neural layer of the retina. It thickens and differentiates into several cellular layers, like the walls of the cerebral vesicles (fig. 1). This differentiation ends by the 7th month. From this time on, the eye is sensitive to light. However, the fovea centralis does not differentiate until 4 months after birth.

2. *Development of the optic stalk*: the optic nerve. — Towards the 7th week the optic stalk forms, encircling the hyaloid artery (fig. 1). The axons of the ganglionic cells progressively colonize it, forming the optic nerve. The axons progress toward the diencephalon and cross over, forming the optic chiasma. From here the fibers reach the specialized structures of the CNS corresponding to the visual sensory system, the external geniculate bodies, and the occipital optic area of the cortex.

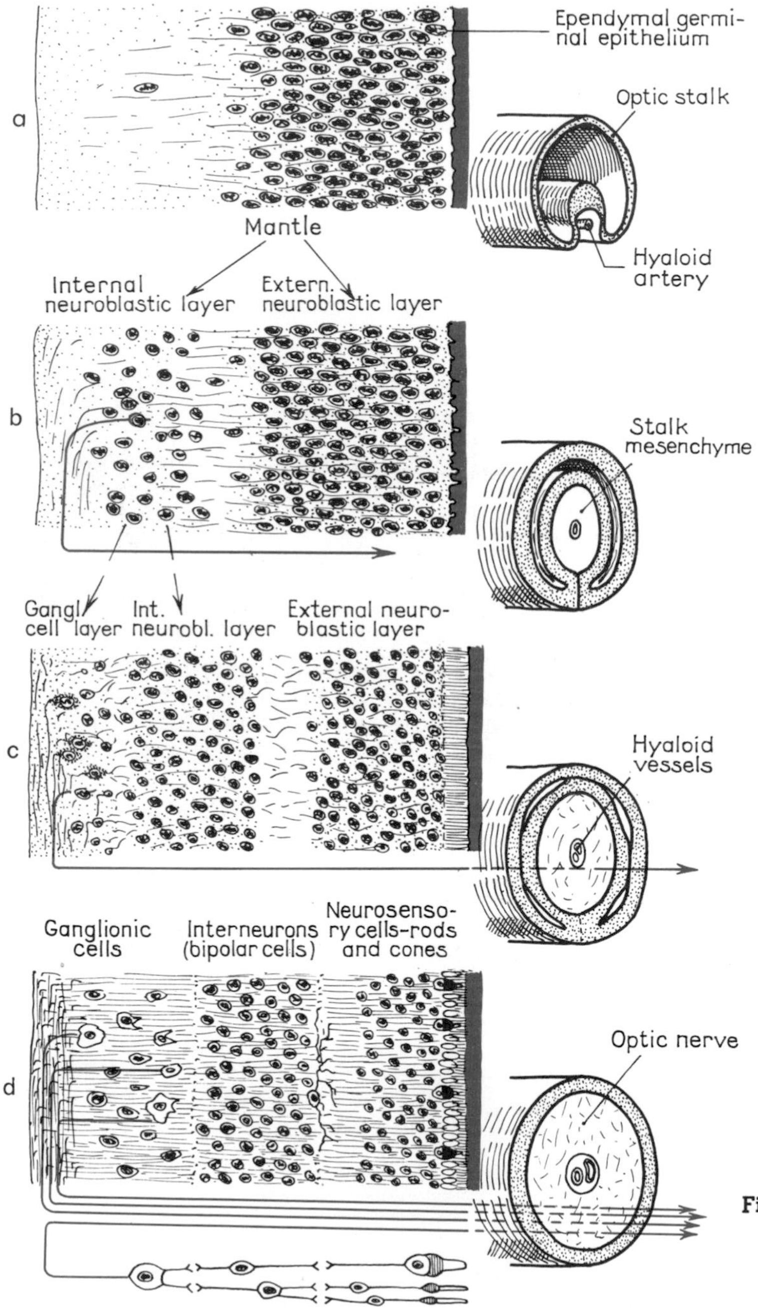

Fig. 1. — *Histogenesis of the human optic retina.* (According to MANN.)

a) about 40 days; *b)* about 45 days; *c)* about 130 days; *d)* about 175 days.

OPTIC VESICLE

3. *Development of the anterior region of the secondary optic vesicle* : **pars iridica retinae.** — The optic vesicle tends to close in front of the lens. An opening is thus delimited, the pupillary orifice (fig. 2 and 4). Here the internal and external layers of the retina unite. The first, which remains thin and does not undergo sensory differentiation here, gives rise to the internal, nonpigmented layer of the iris. The second produces the pigmented epithelium (fig. 4).

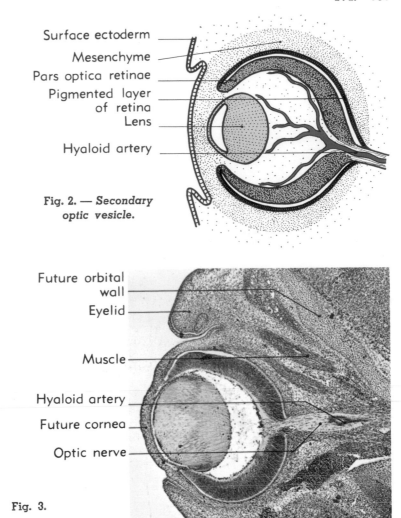

Fig. 2. — *Secondary optic vesicle.*

Surface ectoderm
Mesenchyme
Pars optica retinae
Pigmented layer of retina
Lens
Hyaloid artery

Future orbital wall
Eyelid
Muscle
Hyaloid artery
Future cornea
Optic nerve

Fig. 3.
Eye of a human fetus of about 55 days (× 40).

4. *Ciliary bodies.* — Behind the iris, the two joined retinal layers show several folds containing mesenchyme (fig. 4). These are the ciliary bodies, analagous to the choroid plexes since they secrete the aqueous humor. Between the ciliary folds and the lens, loose fibers form a slender ligament, the suspensor ligament of the lens.

Fig. 4. — *Eye of a human fetus of about 5 months.* The pigmented and neural layers of the retina are shown diagrammatically as separated from each other.

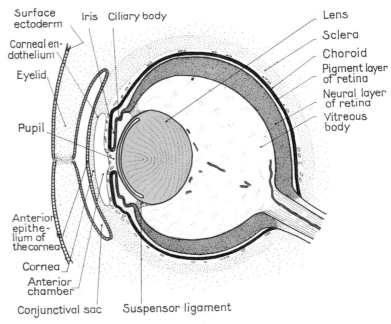

Surface ectoderm
Corneal endothelium
Eyelid
Pupil
Anterior epithelium of the cornea
Cornea
Anterior chamber
Conjunctival sac
Iris
Ciliary body
Suspensor ligament
Lens
Sclera
Choroid
Pigment layer of retina
Neural layer of retina
Vitreous body

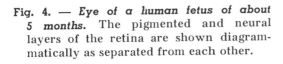

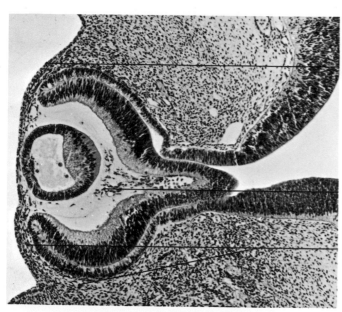

Surface
ectoderm

Primary
vitreous
body

Periocular
mesen-
chyme

Fig. 1. — *Ocular primordium
of a human fetus of about 40 days* (× 100).

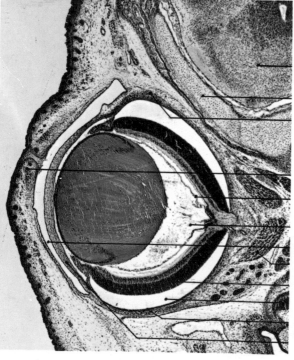

Brain

Bony wall
of orbit
Sclera

Eyelids

Artery of
the retina
Secondary
vitreous body
Conjunctival sac
Muscle

Internal layer
Intraretinal space

External layer
Cornea

Fig. 2. — *Eye of 18-day rat fetus* (× 30). Corresponds to development of about 5 months in man. The space between the external and internal retinal layers is an artifact.

The vitreous body. — The mesenchyme running along the inferior face of the optic primordium invades the optic fissure and fills the optic cup behind the lens. Here it forms the primary vitreous body, which is vascularized by the hyaloid artery (fig. 1).

When the optic fissure is formed about the 7th week, the mesenchyme of the optic stalk is separated from the exterior mesenchyme. The intravesicular portion of the hyaloid artery regresses, while its intra-stalk portion becomes the central artery of the retina. The mesenchymal primary vitreous body then gives rise to an acellular jelly, the secondary vitreous body which fills the optic cup behind the lens (fig. 2 and 3).

Protective coats of the eye. — The protective coats of the eye are derived from the mesenchyme surrounding the optic vesicle.

The choroid is analogous to the pia mater. It is derived from the highly vascularized mesenchyme immediately adjacent to the retina. It provides the conjunctival portion of the iris lining the pars iridica retinae anteriorly (fig. 3).

The sclera is analogous to the dura mater. It is formed by condensation of the peripheral mesenchyme and continues with the sheath of the optic nerve.

OF THE EYE

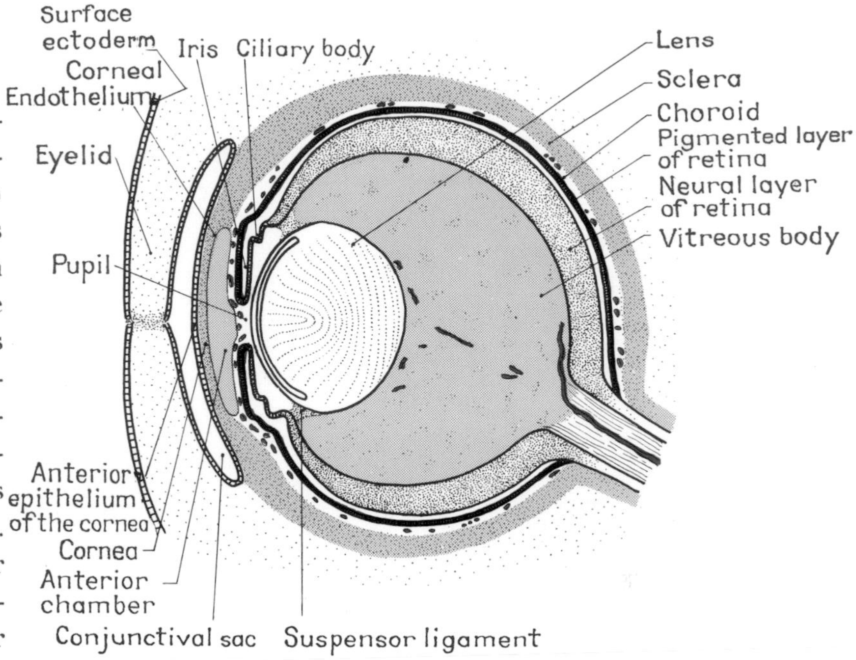

The cornea. — Anteriorly the mesenchyme invades between the surface ectoderm and the lens (fig. 1). It is joined to the surface ectoderm and is continuous with the sclera and gives rise to the cornea (fig. 2 and 3). Under the inductive influence of the lens vesicle and optic vesicle, this mesenchyme undergoes a specific differentiation which makes it perfectly transparent. The adjacent surface ectoderm undergoes an analogous differentiation and forms the anterior epithelium of the cornea (fig.3). Finally, the cornea shows, from the exterior to the interior: a covering of surface ectoderm, the corneal tissue itself, and a layer of flattened mesenchymal cells forming the corneal endothelium.

Multiplication of the mesenchymal cells is such that curvature of the cornea in relation to the sclera is accentuated. This curvature assures basic convergence, and aids the lens in focusing light rays on the retina.

Fig. 3.

Anterior and posterior chambers of the eye. — Because of its curvature, the cornea separates from the subjacent choroid. The space thus formed is the anterior chamber of the eye, limited posteriorly by the corneal epithelium which is curled back on the iris (fig. 3). This endothelium and the choroid form a membrane which covers the pupil during fetal life. Normally this membrane regresses before birth. The posterior chamber forms between the iris and the lens, by progressive separation of these two structures.

The muscles. — The motor muscles of the eyeball (fig. 2) are derived from the peripheral mesenchyme, as well as the ciliary muscles which are involved in convergence of the lens. In contrast, the dilator and constrictor muscles of the iris are derived from the pigmented layer of the iris. These smooth muscles are of ectodermal origin.

The lacrymal glands. — The lacrymal glands are derived from small epithelial cords which penetrate the mesenchyme from the superoexternal area of the conjunctival sac (fig. 2). During the 5th month, these cords give rise to the acini of the definitive gland. The lacrymal duct results from isolation of a cord of surface ectoderm after the convergence of the frontal prominences. Later, this solid cord hollows out.

The eyelids. — The eyelids are simple cutaneous folds, closed at first, which separate about the 7th month. Their morphogenesis is completely independent of that of the eye.

Gross malformations of the eye are formed during the period of organogenesis, that is, between the 20th and the 60th day. However, the eye is still vulnerable to teratogenic agents after this period, especially at the time of histogenesis.

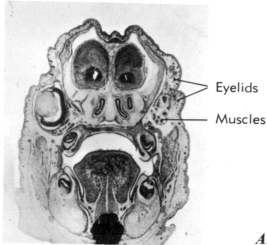

Fig. 1. — *Unilateral anophthalmia.*

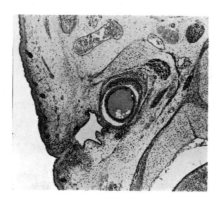

Fig. 2. — *Microphthalmia.*

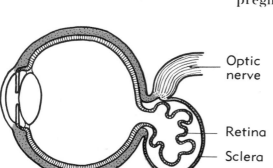

Fig. 3. — *Retinocele.*

I. — DISORDERS OF BASIC ORGANOGENESIS

Cyclopia. — Cyclopia is the presence of a single median eye or two eyes more or less fused on the midline. This condition is never a single isolated malformation. It is part of a complex syndrome associating cyclocephalus and arhinencephalus in varying degrees (see Cyclocephalus, p. 87).

Anophthalmia. — Anophthalmia refers to uni- or bilateral absence of the eyes. The eyelids and motor muscles are present, for the origin of these structures is independent of that of the eye. The malformation is often accompanied by other cranio-cerebral anomalies.

Experimentally, anophthalmia can be produced by pantothenic acid deficiency, hypervitaminosis A, hypoglycemia-producing sulfamides, and other agents.

Microphthalmia. — In microphthalmia the eyeball and the lens are small and more or less malformed. There is frequent association of coloboma. Experimentally, microphthalmia and anophthalmia can be produced by the same methods. In man, the etiology of these malformations is still uncertain. Some cases have been noted after therapeutic irradiation during the first weeks of pregnancy. In certain instances a genetic origin seems probable.

Retinocele. — Retinocele is a herniation of the retina into the sclera, caused by failure of the optic fissure to close. If the hernia is severe, it can cause protrusion of the eyeball.

MALFORMATIONS

Congenital cataract. — In congenital cataract, the structure of the lens is altered and opaque. Experimentally, cataract can be produced by administering chemicals or drugs (thyroxine, for example) to the mother.

In man, rubella, certain other viral infections, and toxoplasmosis are frequent causes, when they are contracted by the mother during the first two months of pregnancy. Other cases are of genetic origin.

Coloboma. — Coloboma represents persistence of the optic fissure after the 7th week. The coloboma may involve the retina and the iris. The cause is unknown. Problems of vision vary according to the severity of the malformation.

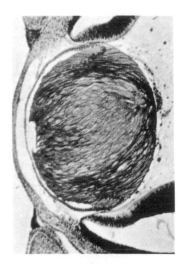

Fig. 4. — *Congenital cataract.*

II. — SECONDARY DISORDERS

Congenital glaucoma. — Congential glaucoma is due to a problem of venous circulation, usually in relation to dysgenesis of the venous system circumscribing the iris. Experimentally, it can be produced by administration of glucagon to the pregnant rat.

Incomplete regression of the hyaloid artery. — This malformation causes problems of vision only if the remnants of the artery are considerable.

Persistence of the pupillary membrane. — This malformation causes only minor problems.

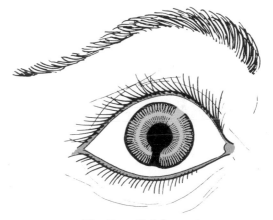

Fig. 5. — *Coloboma.*

Anomalies of eye dimensions. — Such anomalies may be the cause of myopia (optic axis too long) or hyperopia (optic axis too short).

An irregularity of curvature of the cornea or lens causes astigmatism.

Retrolental fibroplasia. — Retrolental fibroplasia is fibrosis of the vitreous body with folding of the retina. It can be produced experimentally by vitamin A deficiency or hyperoxygenation.

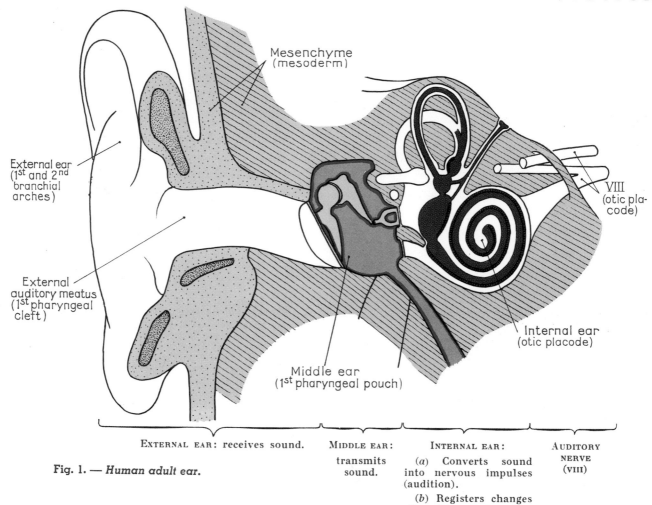

External ear
(1st and 2nd
branchial
arches)

External
auditory meatus
(1st pharyngeal
cleft)

Mesenchyme
(mesoderm)

VIII
(otic pla-
code)

Internal ear
(otic placode)

Middle ear
(1st pharyngeal pouch)

EXTERNAL EAR: receives sound.	MIDDLE EAR: transmits sound.	INTERNAL EAR: (a) Converts sound into nervous impulses (audition). (b) Registers changes of position (balance).	AUDITORY NERVE (VIII)

Fig. 1. — *Human adult ear.*

Development of the ear, the complex organ of hearing and balance, involves the three embryonic germ layers:

— *the ectoderm* is the origin of the internal and external ears;

— *the entoderm* participates in formation of the middle ear;

— *the mesoderm* participates in formation of all three parts of the ear.

Both in phylogenesis and in ontogenesis, the internal ear appears first. In fish, only the internal ear occurs. The middle and external ears do not appear until the amphibians. The three parts of the ear have been improved in the course of evolution. In birds the cochlea is particularly elongated. It is spiral-shaped only in mammals.

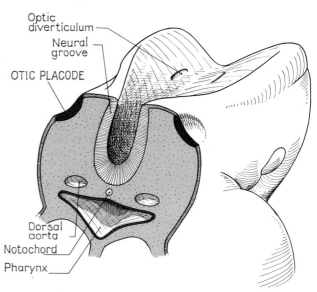

Optic
diverticulum

Neural
groove

OTIC PLACODE

Dorsal
aorta

Notochord

Pharynx

Fig. 2 a. — *About 22 days* (2.5 mm).

SYSTEM

In the human embryo, the auditory placode appears toward the 3rd week in the rhombencephalic region. Primary induction comes from the anterior chordomesoderm and secondarily from the rhombencephalon.

Since cellular proliferation is more intense internally than externally, the placode gradually invaginates. Thus the auditory vesicle is formed, isolated from the superficial ectoderm by its active invagination and by the thrust of the lateral mesenchyme (fig. 2 and 3).

In 50 days, this simple vesicle gives rise to the basic structure of the inner ear. The liquid it contains is found in all its derivatives. This is the endolymphatic fluid, furnished by specific vessels adjacent to the epithelium (fig. 3).

The statoacoustic ganglion cells arise from the inferior internal face of the vesicle. Their dendrites are in contact with the sensory structures of the inner ear and their axons conduct the impulses toward the CNS.

Fig. 3. — *Auditory vesicle of a human embryo of about 28 days* ($\times$ 170).

Fig. 2 a, b, c. — *Cephalic ends of a human embryo, transversaly cut at level of otic placode.*

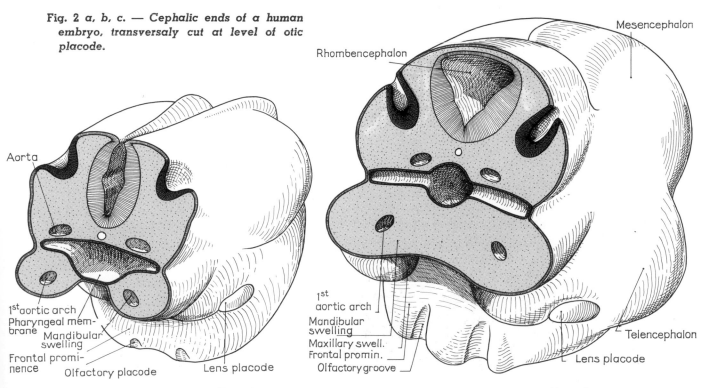

Fig. 2 b. — *About 24 days* (3 mm).

Fig. 2 c. — *About 27 days* (4 mm).

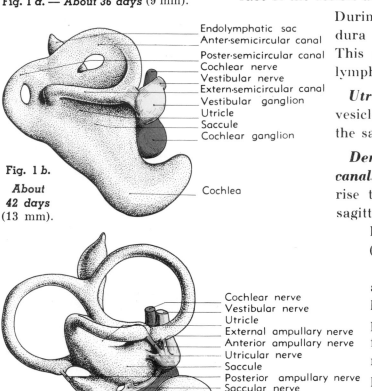

Fig. 1 a. — About 36 days (9 mm).

Endolymphatic sac
Utricular primordium
Vestibular ganglion (Scarpa)
Primordium of anterior semicircular canal
Cochlear ganglion (Corti)
Primordium of saccule

Fig. 1 b.
About 42 days (13 mm).

Endolymphatic sac
Anter·semicircular canal
Poster·semicircular canal
Cochlear nerve
Vestibular nerve
Extern·semicircular canal
Vestibular ganglion
Utricle
Saccule
Cochlear ganglion
Cochlea

Fig. 1 c.
About 50 days (20 mm).

Cochlear nerve
Vestibular nerve
Utricle
External ampullary nerve
Anterior ampullary nerve
Utricular nerve
Saccule
Posterior ampullary nerve
Saccular nerve
Cochlea

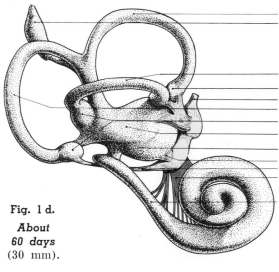

Fig. 1 d.
About 60 days (30 mm).

Anter·semicircular canal
Endolymphatic sac
External semicircular canal
Ampulla
Vestibular nerve
Poster·semicircular canal
Ampullae
UTRICLE } VESTIBULE
SACCULE
Saccular nerve
Posterior ampullar nerve
Cochlear nerve
Cochlea

Fig. 1 a to d.
Development of the membranous labyrinth in man.

I. — DEVELOPMENT OF THE AUDITORY VESICLE

The membranous labyrinth is formed from derivatives of the auditory vesicle.

Endolymphatic duct or sac. — The endolymphatic sac is an evagination which appears about the 30th day on the internal face of the vesicle and which gradually elongates dorsally (fig. 1 a). During the second half of pregnancy it reaches the dura mater across the surrounding mesenchyme. This duct plays a role in resorption of the endolymphatic fluid.

Utricle and saccule. — The primary auditory vesicle constricts, forming the utricle dorsally and the saccule ventrally (fig. 1 a).

Derivatives of the utricle: the semicircular canals. — The external half of the utricle gives rise to two flat evaginations. One is vertical and sagittal with respect to the embryo, the other is horizontal with its apex toward the exterior (fig. 1 b).

The vertical primordium gives rise to the anterior and posterior vertical canals, back to back, according to the axis of evagination. The primordium of the anterior canal differentiates first about the 36th day. Its central portion is rapidly resorbed, thus forming the canal. The posterior primordium undergoes the same development after several hours. The common median portion of the two primordia persists in the form of the common trunk of the two canals (fig. 1 b, c, and d).

The horizontal primordium, perpendicular to the first two, undergoes the same development after 3 or 4 days. Morphogenesis of these three canals is complete about the 50th day.

One of the ends of each canal opens into the utricle by a swelling, the ampulla, where the sensory organ of balance develops (fig. 1 d and 2, the crista).

The final transformation of the system consists of a 90° displacement of the anterior canal to the outside. The three canals are thus placed in the three planes of space. They will now show only an increase in size, until the 6th month.

THE INTERNAL EAR

Derivatives of the saccule: the cochlea.

About the 36th day, the saccule shows a ventral evagination which progressively elongates. It is straight at first, but soon spirals because of unequal growth of the external and internal faces (fig. 1). By the 70th day of gestation, the cochlea has 2½ spiral turns. Its morphogenesis is finished.

II. — DEVELOPMENT OF PERIPHERAL MESENCHYME

Osseous labyrinth.

At some distance from the membranous labyrinth, the peripheral mesenchyme becomes organized into cartilage towards the 5th week, and begins to form bone after the 8th week (otic capsule) (fig. 2). Several islets of cartilage may persist after birth. If they hypertrophy, they may play a role in the formation of otospongiosis.

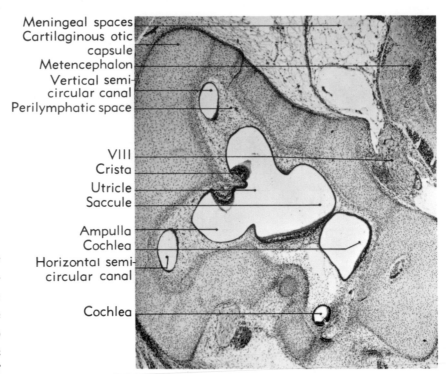

Meningeal spaces
Cartilaginous otic capsule
Metencephalon
Vertical semi-circular canal
Perilymphatic space

VIII
Crista
Utricle
Saccule

Ampulla
Cochlea
Horizontal semi-circular canal

Cochlea

Fig. 2. — *Frontal section of the inner ear in a human fetus of about 70 days* ($\times$ 30).

Perilymphatic spaces.

The perilymphatic spaces are derived from the mesenchyme between the membranous and the osseous labyrinths (fig. 2). While the latter differentiates, the mesenchyme is transformed into a large-meshed reticulum containing a fluid, the perilymph.

The perilymphatic spaces corresponding to the cochlea are divided into a vestibular, suprachoclear space, the scala vestibuli, and a subcochlear tympanic space, the scala tympani (fig. 4, p. 111).

These two spaces are independent, for mesenchymal resorption is not complete. Outside, the mesenchyme gives rise to the spiral ligament and inside, a bony plate, the spiral plate (fig. 3 and 4, p. 111). These two spaces are united only at the end of the cochlea through a small orifice which forms in the spiral plate at the end of the 3rd month.

The perilymphatic spaces are connected with the meningeal spaces by a fine duct, the cochlear duct, which runs through the otic capsule opposite the saccule. Resorption of the perilymph occurs through this pathway.

III. — FORMATION OF THE NEURAL SENSORY FIBERS

The ganglionic cells derived from the placode are grouped into two clusters. One, the ganglion of Scarpa, is joined to the vestibular portion of the labyrinth. The other is joined to the cochlear duct; this is the ganglion of Corti (fig. 1). The dendrites of these cells reach the sensory epithelium of the inner ear. The axons progress toward the metencephalon, bunching together to form the acoustic nerve (8th cranial nerve). After metencephalic connections (nuclei of VIII), the vestibular fibers reach the cerebellum (subconscious balance) and the cochlear fibers reach the internal geniculate body, then the temporal cortex (conscious sound sensations).

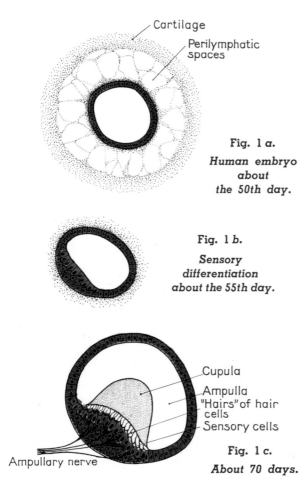

Cartilage
Perilymphatic spaces

Fig. 1 a.

Human embryo about the 50th day.

Fig. 1 b.

Sensory differentiation about the 55th day.

Cupula
Ampulla
"Hairs" of hair cells
Sensory cells

Ampullary nerve

Fig. 1 c.

About 70 days.

Fig. 1 a, b, c. — Sections of the ampulla
of one of the semicircular canals
at various stages.

I. — HISTOGENESIS OF THE SEMICIRCULAR CANALS

The columnar epithelium lining the auditory vesicle and its derivatives flattens, except in the regions of the ampullae (fig. 1 a, b, and fig. 2, p. 109). There, toward the 50th day, the cells take on sensory characteristics under the influence of the dendrites coming from the associated ganglion (Scarpa). At their apical pole, they produce:

— *the hair cells;*

— *the gelatinous mass of the cupula* resting on the hair cells. The cupula is thus mobile. During rotation of the head there is displacement of the endolymph which excites the sensory cells. The cells, their flagella (hairs), and the cupula form the crista, which is completely differentiated around the 70th day of gestation (fig. 1 c).

Analogous organs, the maculae, differentiate in the utricle and the saccule. Here the sensory hairs are covered by a gelatinous mass, the otolithic membrane. On its free surface are calcified structures, the otoliths. The maculae are sensitive to linear acceleration.

II. — HISTOGENESIS OF THE COCHLEA

1. Epithelial derivatives

About the 70th day, the ventral face of the cochlear tube thickens (fig. 2). Cellular proliferations especially involve the external and internal areas separated by a small depression, the spiral sulcus.

The tectorial membrane, gelatinous and fibrous, is derived from the internal portion or spiral limbus (fig. 2 and 3).

The organ of Corti is derived from the external portion. Between the 3rd and the 5th months, certain epithelial cells give rise to ciliated inner and outer sensory cells. The intermediary epithelial cells give rise to various categories of supporting cells (fig. 3 and 4). Here also, sensory differentiation seems to require the presence of dendrites from the associated ganglion (of Corti). In the 5th month, fissures in these groups of cells appear. One forms the spiral sulcus which then clearly separates the organ of Corti from the limbus (fig. 4). Another produces the canal of Corti which isolates the inner ciliated cells from the outer ciliated cells.

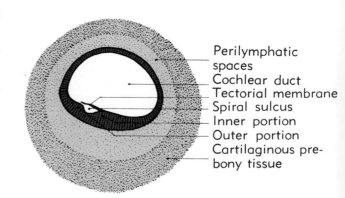

Perilymphatic spaces
Cochlear duct
Tectorial membrane
Spiral sulcus
Inner portion
Outer portion
Cartilaginous pre-bony tissue

Fig. 2. — Human embryo of about 70 days.

THE INTERNAL EAR

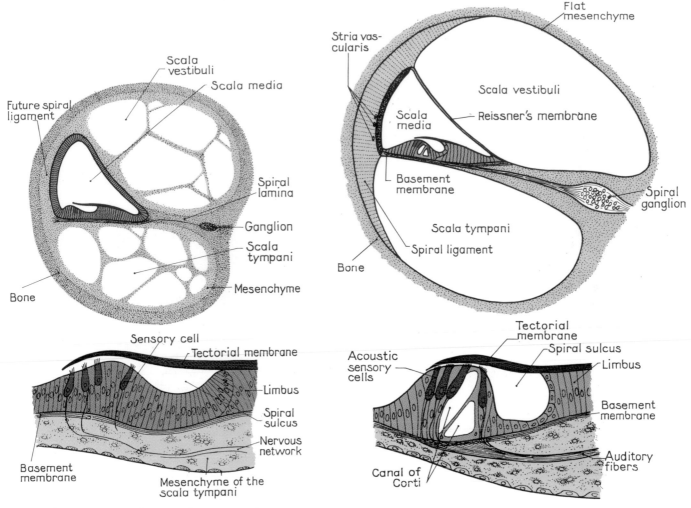

Fig. 3. — *Human embryo of about 5 months.*

Fig. 4. — *At term.*

Reissner's membrane is derived from the dorsal face of the cochlear tube. It remains unstratified and becomes very thin.

The external face of the tube has a thicker epithelium and numerous vessels (stria vascularis). These produce the endolymphatic fluid (fig. 4).

2. *Membranous derivatives*

The fibrillar basement membrane is derived from the mesenchyme lining the ventral face of the organ of Corti (fig. 3 and 4). It is inserted on the ligament and the spiral lamina. It is lined by the mesenchymal lamina bordering the scala tympani (fig. 3).

Histogenesis of the cochlea is complete at 6 months.

3. *Function of the principal derivatives*

When vibrations reach the scala tympani (fig. 3, p. 114), the basement membrane is distorted. This produces movement in the sensory cells whose apical hairs stroke the tectorial membrane, exciting the nerve endings.

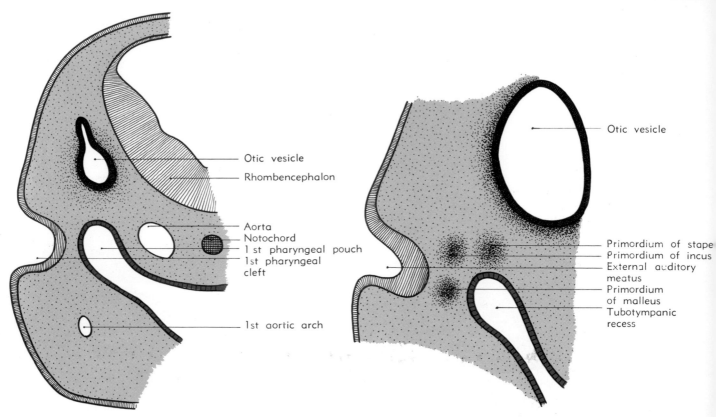

Fig. 1. — *Human embryo of about 50 days.*

Fig. 2. — *Human embryo of about 2 months.*

The middle ear is derived from the first pharyngeal pouch. This pouch gives rise to the epithelia of the Eustachian tube and the tympanic cavity as well as the cavities of the mastoid (fig. 1).

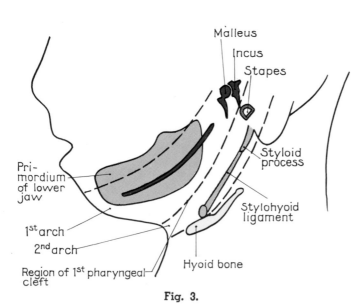

Fig. 3.

The tympanic cavity is formed by the dorsal portion of the pouch which grows in the direction of the external auditory meatus (EAM). At the end of the 6th month, the external wall of the tympanic cavity comes into contact with the deep end of the EAM. A thin mesodermic plate persists between the ectodermal and endodermal epithelial structures; the combination is the eardrum (fig. 1 and 5).

The ossicles differentiate during the 2nd month from mesenchyme neighboring the tympanic cavity (fig. 2 and 6). The cartilage of the 2nd branchial arch, Reichert's cartilage, gives rise first to the stapes, then the cartilage of the 1st arch, Meckel's cartilage, gives rise to the incus and the malleus (fig. 3 and 4).

EAR

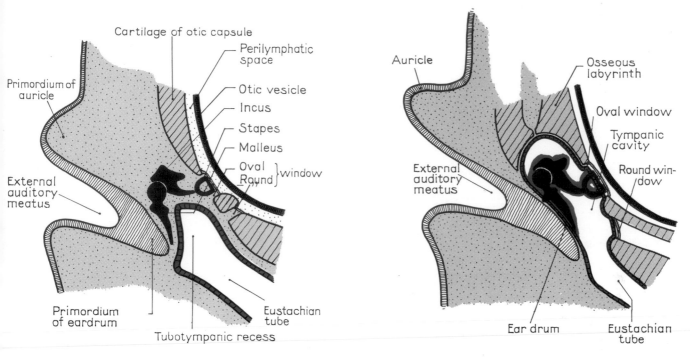

Fig. 4. — *Human fetus of about 3 months.*

Fig. 5. — *Fetus of about 6 months.*

Because of their progressive enlargement, the walls of the tympanic cavity are pushed against the ossicles. These bones therefore project into the interior of the cavity (fig. 5).

At birth, the cavities of the middle ear fill with air through the Eustachian tube. With the ossicles, they form the system used for transmitting vibrations to the inner ear (fig. 5).

The portion of the osseous labyrinth opposite the stapes remains very thin. This is the oval window opening into the scala vestibuli. Below this another thinning of the bony labyrinth forms the round window opening into the scala tympani (fig. 4 and 5) (See *Summary of Function*, p. 114).

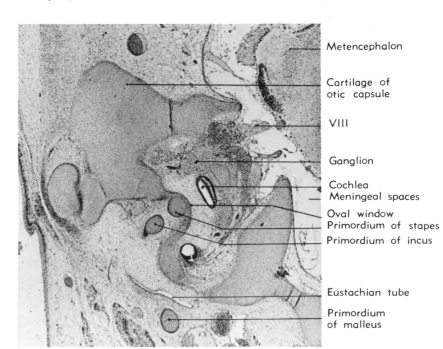

Fig. 6. — *Frontal section of ear of a human fetus of about 70 days* ($\times$ 20).

EXTERNAL EAR

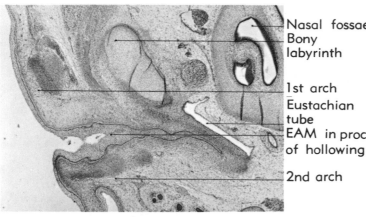

Nasal fossae
Bony labyrinth

1st arch
Eustachian tube
EAM in process of hollowing

2nd arch

Fig. 1. — Frontal section of ear of a human fetus of about 70 days (× 27).

The external ear is derived from the dorsal portion of the first branchial groove and the external covering of the 1st and 2nd arches which border it (fig. 1).

This groove gives rise to a massive cellular cord through proliferation of the surface ectoderm. The cord reaches the tympanic cavity, and later hollows out to form the external auditory meatus (EAM, fig. 1).

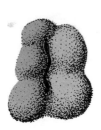
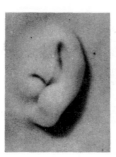
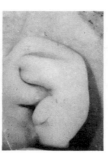
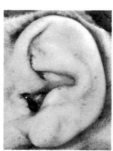
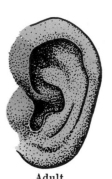

Human embryo of 13 mm: about 42 days.

40 mm: about 65 days.

52 mm: about 72 days.

135 mm: about 4½ months.

Adult.

Fig. 2. — The auricle is formed by the coalescence of small tubercules which appear around the upper part of the branchial groove about the 40th day. The anterior tubercules (dark pink) are derived from the mandibular side of the first branchial groove, and the posterior (light pink) from the hyoid side. The external ear is practically finished about the 4th month.

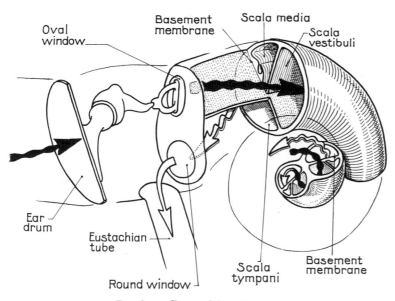

Oval window

Basement membrane

Scala media

Scala vestibuli

Ear drum

Eustachian tube

Round window

Scala tympani

Basement membrane

Fig. 3. — General function.

Summary of function

The elastic *oval window* allows transmission of vibrations to the perilymphatic fluid, then to the basement membrane. The equally elastic *round window* allows for decompression of the system.

The basement membrane acts like a frequency analyzer. It is sensitive to high frequencies toward its base, and low frequencies toward its summit. In marsupials, where final development takes place outside of the uterus, it has been shown that sensitivity of the ear to low frequencies corresponds with progressive elongation of the cochlea.

MALFORMATIONS

Malformations of the auditory system may be classed into three different groups, corresponding to the distinct embryological characteristics of each of the three parts of the ear.

LESIONS OF THE INTERNAL EAR

Cochlea. — Rubella in the 2nd month of pregnancy is frequently a cause of lesions of the cochlea, for this is the period of differentiation of the internal ear. The epithelium of the cochlea and the vestibule is altered. The organ of Corti has some intact regions, so that children affected by this condition may perceive some deep frequencies.

Canals. — Few malformations of the canals are known. However, several cases caused by thalidomide have been reported. Similar lesions are found in waltzing mice, where they are hereditary.

Experimentally, a deficiency of manganese has been found to produce abnormal development of the inner ear in the rat. Malformations of the afferent nerve tract may also result.

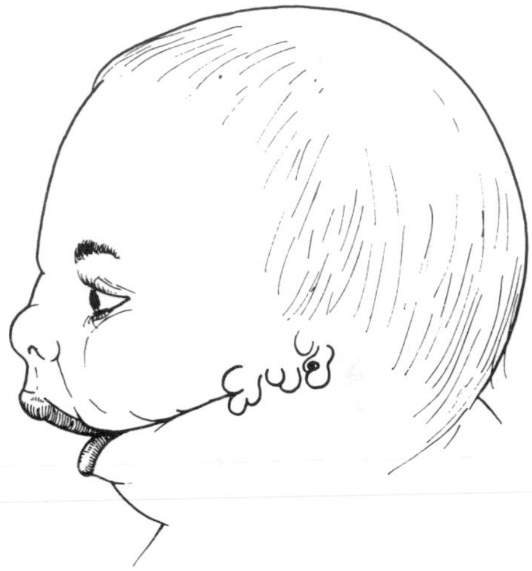

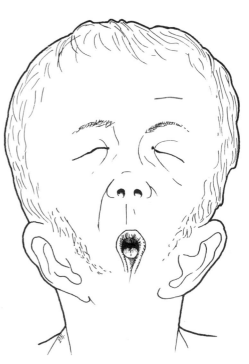

Fig. 4. — *Anomaly of external ear with maxillomandibular fissure.*

LESIONS OF THE MIDDLE EAR

Lesions of the middle ear usually involve the ossicles. Following an infection, for example, the mesenchymal plate which separates the ossicles may become sclerotic and impede their normal movement. This lesion may result in total deafness.

MALFORMATIONS OF THE EXTERNAL EAR

Malformations of the external ear result from absence or nonunion of the tubercles from which it arises. There are also abnormal positions of the ear, usually in relation to a problem of mandibular development, *agnathia or micrognathia*. Instead of moving to the sides of the head, the ears continue to develop at the site of the primordia, that is, at the level of the first branchial groove. They are thus found in the newborn at the angle of the missing jaw. This is *otocephalus,* and is of genetic origin.

Fig. 5. — *Otocephalus, medium type.*

ENDOCRINE GLANDS

NEUROENDOCRINE

Neuroendocrine correlations result from interactions between the endocrine glands and the CNS. These interactions occur through the vascular and nervous systems. They involve a central system, the hypothalamic-hypophyseal combination, and a peripheral system formed by the other endocrine glands (fig. 1).

I. — ACTION OF THE CENTRAL NERVOUS SYSTEM ON THE ENDOCRINE GLANDS

In the adult, the action of the nervous system on the endocrine glands is very important. It occurs through the intermediary of the hypothalamus. Experimentally, stimulation of certain hypothalamic nuclei, or lesions in others, brings about liberation of various trophic hormones from the anterior pituitary. There are thus nervous centers activating and inhibiting the hypophysis. Their action brings about puberty and accounts for estrous cycles in the female. All these processes cease or are greatly decreased if the hypothalamic-hypophyseal connections are interrupted (fig. 2).

Among the numerous factors affecting the hypophysis, many are external. Transmission occurs through the sense organs and the CNS. The hypothalamus responds by liberating hypophyseal stimulants. Some lower vertebrates adapt to the light in their environment in this way by changing their color (liberation of intermedine, see p. 126). Similar mechanisms account for defective spermatogenesis in ducks placed in a dark environment, the seasonal rhythm of gonadotrophic hormone secretion in many mammals, and the fact that a serious emotional shock can affect puberty and ovulation or bring about precocious menopause in women. All these interactions are examples of neurosensory-endocrine integrations.

In the fetus, the action of the CNS on the endocrine glands is more limited. However, normal hypothalamic function seems to be necessary for development of the adrenal cortex (see p. 136).

II. — ACTION OF THE ENDOCRINE GLANDS ON THE CENTRAL NERVOUS SYSTEM

In the adult, there are two types of action of the endocrine glands on the CNS.

a) **Quantitative regulation:** increase in levels of circulating hormones modifies hypothalmic stimulation of the anterior pituitary. To a lesser degree, it may also directly repress production of hypophyseal hormones.

b) **Qualitative modifications:** presence or absence of hormones in the blood affects the CNS and modifies behavior. Thus, the sex hormones influence sexual behavior, while thyroxine increases excitability. Hydrocortisone maintains the adrenal cortex and the reticular formation at an optimal level of excitability by affecting Na and Ca exchange.

In the fetus, the endocrine glands have an inductive role, for the hormones affect even development of the CNS itself.

a) **Action of thyroid hormone.** — Thyroxin seems to be necessary for the maturation of the CNS, especially for migration of the cortical cells. A congenital insufficiency of the thyroid produces myxedema with mental retardation and behavior problems. Experimentally in the rat, neonatal thyroidectomy causes cessation of growth of cerebral cell bodies and a decrease in their dendrites and axons. At the same time, behavioral development of the animals is retarded. These observations are consistent with the idea that protein synthesis is disturbed because of the thyroid deficiency. Experimental neonatal hyperthyroidism has effects opposite to these and in particular stimulates myelinization. Clinically, some hyperthyroid children show increased emotionality.

CORRELATIONS

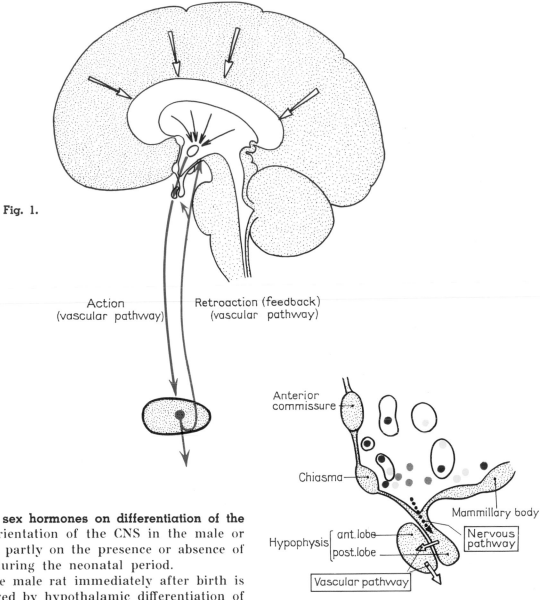

Fig. 1.

Action
(vascular pathway)

Retroaction (feedback)
(vascular pathway)

Anterior
commissure

Chiasma

Mammillary body

Hypophysis { ant. lobe / post. lobe }

Nervous
pathway

Vascular pathway

Fig. 2.

b) **Action of the sex hormones on differentiation of the hypothalamus.** — Orientation of the CNS in the male or female type depends partly on the presence or absence of the male hormone during the neonatal period.

Castration of the male rat immediately after birth is spontaneously followed by hypothalamic differentiation of the female type, while injection of androgens into the female under the same conditions brings about a male differentiation. Thus the role of the androgenic hormones appears to be fundamental in sexual differentiation.

In the female, the adult hypothalamus exerts a rhythmic regulation on the secretion of gonadotrophic hormones so that the ovary has a periodic cycle, with formation of follicles and corpora lutea.

In the male, on the other hand, the hypothalamus maintains secretion of the gonadotrophins at a relatively constant level for non-cyclical sexual activity.

We will study the development of the glands which have specific relationships with the nervous system, the hypophysis, the paraganglia, and the adrenals. The other endocrine glands are dealt with in Volume 2.

DEVELOPMENT

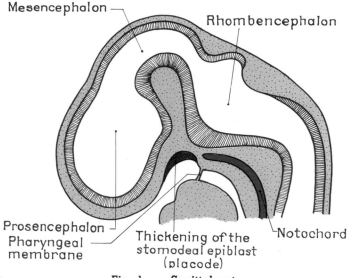

Fig. 1. — *Sagittal cut of cephalic end of an human embryo about 22 days.*

The hypophysis, or pituitary gland, is an unpaired endocrine gland situated in the sella turcica. It is found in all vertebrates. It consists of two parts of different origins. The glandular portion comes from an evagination of the epithelium covering the vault of the stomodeum. The diencephalic neural portion comes from an evagination of the floor of the 3rd ventricle. During embryonic development, the glandular primordium becomes located anterior to the neural primordium (fig. 2).

The glandular primordium is induced first by the anterior end of the notochordal system, perhaps by the prechordal plate (fig. 1). This system next induces the neural primordium or infundibulum. From this time on, each primordium affects development of the other through reciprocal inductions.

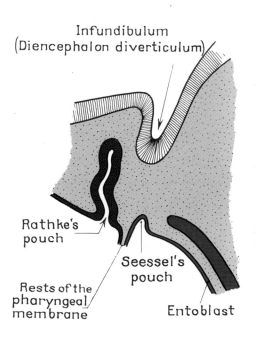

Fig. 2. — *Human embryo about 42 days.*

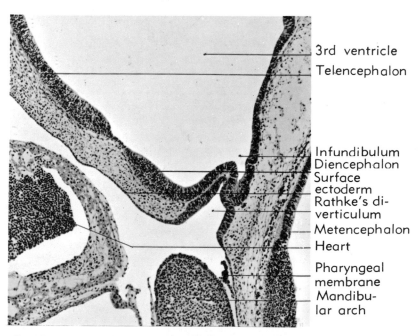

Fig. 3. — *Hypophyseal primordium of a rat fetus of 13 days.* Sagittal section (× 70). The notochord is not visible.

OF THE HYPOPHYSIS

l. — *THE GLANDULAR PRIMORDIUM*

About the 21st day (7 somites) the cells of the stomodeal surface ectoderm just ahead of the pharyngeal membrane become thicker than the others. This placodal primordium is very near the wall of the diencephalon and just ahead of the notochord (fig. 1).

Then the flat primordium invaginates and penetrates the mesenchyme in the direction of the diencephalon ([1]). It thus forms the *diverticulum of Rathke,* then the *pouch of Rathke,* which is flat and situated just ahead of the neural primordium (fig. 2 to 5).

Rathke's pouch is attached to the stomodeal vault by the pharyngohypophyseal stalk, which regresses and disappears at about 1½ months (fig. 4 and 5). Parts of it, however, may persist in a more or less differentiated and sometimes functional condition. These constitute the pharyngeal hypophysis (in the region of invagination) and the sphenoidal or sellar parahypophysis.

Just behind the pharyngeal membrane, the entodermal epithelium also forms a pouch, the pouch of Seessel (fig. 2). This is involved in formation of the glandular hypophysis in lower vertebrates. However, this involvement decreases as the evolutionary scale increases, and disappears completely in primates and man. In man it sometimes persists and is the cause of certain tumors (see p. 129).

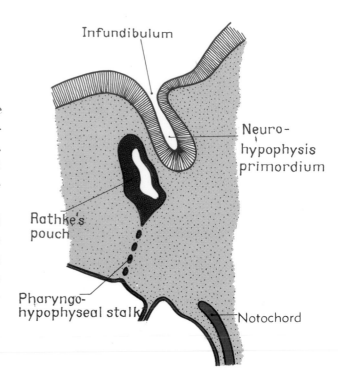

Fig. 4. — *Human fetus about 60 days.*

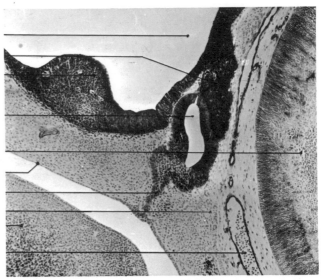

Fig. 5. — *Rat fetus of 15 days.*

([1]) This corresponds to the general development of placodes in vertebrates (p. 94).

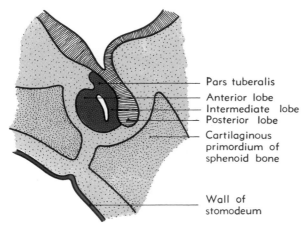

Pars tuberalis
Anterior lobe
Intermediate lobe
Posterior lobe
Cartilaginous primordium of sphenoid bone

Wall of stomodeum

Fig. 1. — *Sagittal section of pituitary of a human fetus of 2 months.*

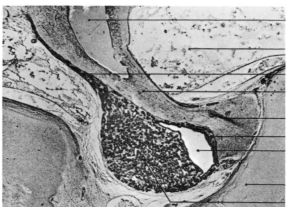

Infundibulum

Meningeal spaces

Pars tuberalis

Pituitary stalk

Posterior lobe

Intermediate lobe
Cavity of Rathke's pouch

Sphenoid

Anterior lobe

Fig. 2. — *Pituitary of a human fetus of about 2 1/2 months.* Sagittal section (× 15).

1. Development of the anterior wall of Rathke's pouch

The anterior lobe or adenohypophysis. — The anterior wall proliferates activly. The cellular columns anastomose within the surrounding mesenchyme and produce the anterior lobe of the hypophysis (fig. 1 and 2). Proliferation occurs in such a way that a small basin is formed, open above and separated into 2 compartments by a median cellular septum. Each compartment, or fossa of Atwell, is filled with mesenchyme. The fossae disappear progressively due to parietal growth. The median septum forms the pars medialis, and the lateral portions form the pars lateralis of the anterior lobe (fig. 3).

Morphogenesis of the anterior lobe of the hypophysis thus shows bilateral symmetry.

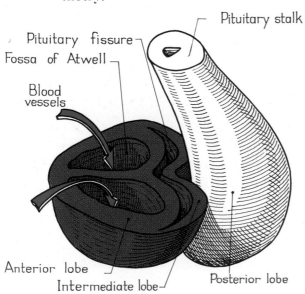

Pituitary stalk

Pituitary fissure
Fossa of Atwell

Blood vessels

Anterior lobe
Intermediate lobe
Posterior lobe

The pars tuberalis. — The median septum proliferates upward along the pituitary stalk, which is gradually encircled by the cellular expansion of the developing pars tuberalis (fig. 1, 2, and 4).

Fig. 3. — *Cross section of pituitary of a human fetus of 2 months.*

RATHKE'S POUCH

Histogenesis. — Histogenesis begins about the 4th month. The glandular character of the differentiation seems to be induced by the surrounding mesenchyme. Cellular differentiation occurs from the same cellular layer. The cells reflect the bilateral symmetry noted during morphogenesis. The basophil (or PAS+) cells are much more numerous in the anteromedian than in the posterolateral areas, while the acidophils (or PAS−−) show the opposite location (fig. 5). These localizations correspond to the secretion of different hormones. The chromophobe cells are spread almost uniformly, for chromophobia characterizes: *a*) the phase of hyperactivity of various cellular categories, with rapid emptying of the products of secretion, and *b*) absence of secretory activity in the undifferentiated cell layers.

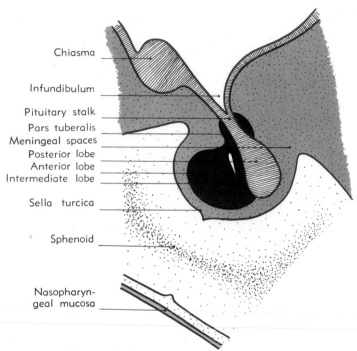

Fig. 4. — *Sagittal section of pituitary of a human fetus of 3 months.*

2. *Development of the posterior wall of Rathke's pouch*

The intermediate lobe. — The posterior wall develops very little in man. It gives rise to the intermediate lobe or pars intermedia, joined to the neural lobe (fig. 1 to 5). Its cells progressively invade the anterior lobe and by puberty the intermediate lobe has more or less disappeared.

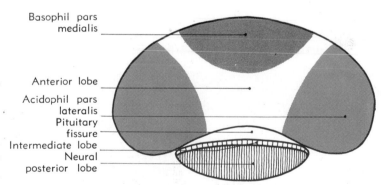

Fig. 5. — *Cross section of adult pituitary*: relative density of acidophilic and basophilic cells is shown (according to GIROUD and DESCLAUX).

3. *Development of the cavity of Rathke's pouch*

In man, growth of the walls of the pouch makes this cavity extremely narrow. This is the pituitary fissure. It is effaced by progressive incorporation of cells from the intermediate and anterior lobes.

II. — NEURAL PRIMORDIUM

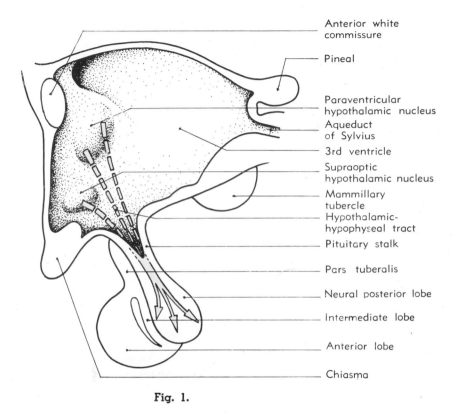

Anterior white
commissure

Pineal

Paraventricular
hypothalamic nucleus

Aqueduct
of Sylvius

3rd ventricle

Supraoptic
hypothalamic nucleus

Mammillary
tubercle

Hypothalamic-
hypophyseal tract

Pituitary stalk

Pars tuberalis

Neural posterior lobe

Intermediate lobe

Anterior lobe

Chiasma

Fig. 1.

About the 40th day, a little behind the glandular primordium, the floor of the 3rd ventricle is depressed and produces the infundibulum (fig. 2, p. 120). This depression penetrates progressively toward the glandular primordium, and about the 45th day its ventral end forms a diverticulum. This structure thickens and its lumen gradually fills. This is the neural lobe which is attached to the posterior wall of Rathke's pouch. It remains attached to the diencephalon by a thin stalk, the pituitary or hypophyseal stalk (fig. 1). The infundibulum, the stalk, and the posterior lobe form the neural hypophysis.

During the 4th month, the neural lobe differentiates and specific neuroglial cells appear, the pituicytes. Some investigators believe these cells to be glandular, but this has not been proved.

The neurohypophysis is then colonized by axons coming from the hypothalamic nuclei (fig. 1). These axons form the hypothalamic-hypophyseal tract, the pathway for hypothalamic neurosecretion. Rich in polypeptides, this is elaborated in the hypothalamic nuclei by cells which appear to be both neural and glandular (paraventricular and supraoptic nuclei among others).

The neurosecretory material (NSM) is conducted to the neurohypophysis by the axons of these cells, and may be discerned in the fetus at about 4 months (fig. 2).

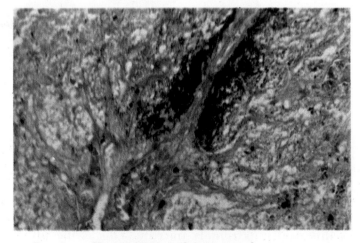

Fig. 2. — *Neurosecretion demonstrated in the neural lobe of a human fetus of about 6 months. In violet,* neurosecretion granules. *In blue,* fibers of the hypothalamo - hypophyseal tract (stained with hematoxylin-paraldehyde-fuchsin).

III. — RELATIONSHIPS BETWEEN NEURAL AND GLANDULAR HYPOPHYSIS

A certain portion of the neurosecretion passes from the hypothalamus to the glandular hypophysis where it regulates production of the various trophic hormones. This is accomplished through the blood via a "portal" system in the following way:

The superior hypophyseal arteries (fig. 3) arise from the internal carotid and form a capillary bed in the proximal half of the neurohypophysis. These capillaries collect the neurosecretory material (NSM) (fig. 3 *b*). The venules which follow them pass into the pars tuberalis and the anterior lobe (fig. 3 *c* and *d*) where they resolve into a new capillary system which releases the NSM.

The particular arrangement constitutes the **portal system** of the hypophysis (fig. 3 *d*: portal vein). It represents the essential pathway of neuroadenohypophyseal relationships. The following experiment demonstrates this system. If the anterior lobe of a rat is removed from the neural portion and grafted on another part of the organism, it shows no reduction of activity. If it is reimplanted in the subhypothalamic space, it is revascularized by capillaries of the portal system and seems to recover its normal functions (Harris and Jacobsohn).

The inferior hypophyseal arteries (fig. 3 *e*) come from the internal carotids. They irrigate the neural lobe and do not seem to be connected with the portal system. The veins which follow carry the so-called hormones of the posterior lobe, which are really more or less modified neurosecretions, from this lobe.

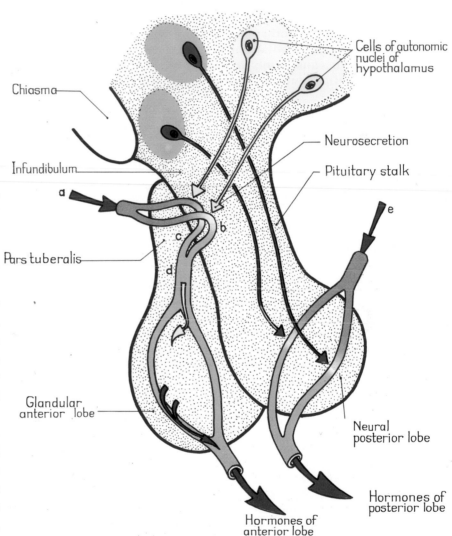

Fig. 3. — *Diagram of neuroadenohypophyseal relationships.*

During the 4th month, differentiation of the anterior and intermediate lobes is accomplished, and neurosecretion of hypothalamic origin appears in the neural lobe. The beginning of physiological activity corresponds to these histological changes, and is marked by stimulation of the thyroid (presence of thyrotrophic hormone in the blood). This activity and the neuroendocrine correlations of the human fetus are very different from those of the adult.

I. — PHYSIOLOGICAL ROLE OF ANTERIOR PITUITARY

After birth and in the adult. — All the endocrine receptors are dependent on hypophyseal stimulation (1).

In the fetus, on the other hand, some endocrine glands partially or completely escape this control. In fact, although experimental ablation of the fetal hypophysis results in severe atrophy of the adrenals and the thyroid, it causes only a slowing of gonadal development. Also, it has been noted that signs of glandular stimulation during the 4th month involve mainly the adrenal cortex and the thyroid (fig. 1, opposite).

In addition, hypophysectomy does not affect fetal growth. In contrast to juvenile growth, fetal growth therefore seems to be independent of growth hormone.

II. — NEUROENDOCRINE CORRELATIONS

In the adult, all the trophic hormones of the anterior pituitary seem to be more or less under control of the hypothalamic nuclei. Actually, NSM includes inhibitory as well as releasing factors which regulate secretion of the various trophic hormones through the hypophyseal portal system (fig. 3, p. 125) (2).

In the fetus, on the other hand, hypothalamic control seems much less important. Only secretion of ACTH requires nervous stimulation, as is suggested by observations in anencephalics (fig. 1, opposite, and see p. 136).

III. — THE INTERMEDIATE LOBE

The intermediate lobe produces the melanotrophic hormone (MSH) or intermedin. This hormone stimulates movement of pigment in the melanophores from the cell body to the cell processes. This phenomenon is especially visible in the skin of fish and amphibians, and is seen in mammals in the pigmented epithelium of the retina.

IV. — HYPOPHYSIS AND CEREBRAL EPIPHYSIS

In the fetus and in the prepuberal child, the epiphysis (pineal) is antagonistic to the gonadotrophic cells of the hypophysis. Its experimental or pathologic (tumor) destruction causes precocious development of the sex organs and secondary sex characteristics. Lesions associated with nervous centers probably play a role in these problems (excitation of the hypothalamic nuclei related to gonadotrophic function). The endocrine role of the epiphysis ceases at puberty.

(1) *Gonadotrophic hormones.* a) Follicle-stimulating hormone or FSH: development of the ovarian follicle and of spermatogenesis.

b) Luteinizing hormone or LH: endocrine activity of the testis after the prenatal period; ovulation and appearance of the ovarian corpus luteum, synergistic with FSH.

c) Prolactin, or lactogenic hormone: in women, postpartum lactation. In the rat this hormone is also necessary for maintenance of progesterone secretion by the corpus luteum of pregnancy.

Thyrotrophic hormone, or TSH.

Somatotrophic or growth hormone, or STH.

Adrenal corticotrophic hormone, or ACTH. Development of the fetal adrenal cortex and primordium of the cortical zone of the definitive cortex (see p. 134).

(2) In the adult, neurosecretion also includes the hormones of the posterior lobe, oxytocin and vasopressin or antidiuretic hormone (ADH) (fig. 3, p. 125), which comes from the supraoptic and paraventricular nuclei.

FETAL HYPOPHYSIS

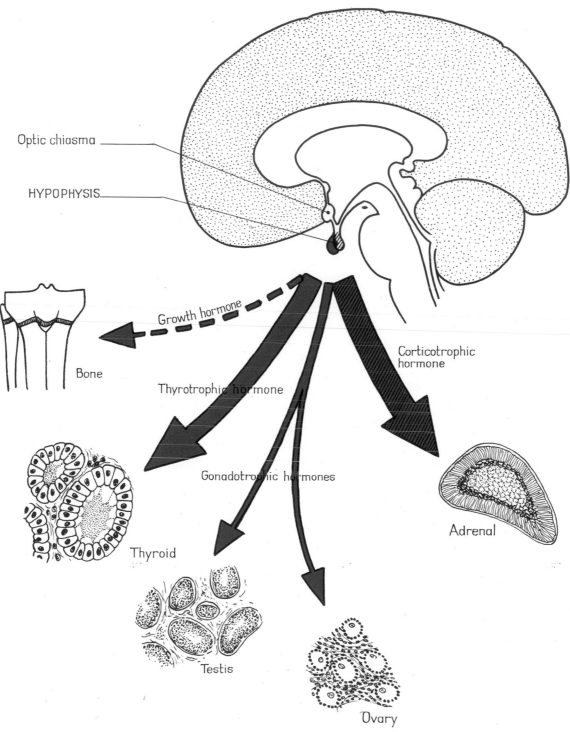

Fig. 1. — *Neuroendocrine correlations during fetal life.* The arrows show independence *(dashed arrow)*, partial dependence *(narrow arrow)*, or total dependence *(wide arrow)* of the endocrine receptors on the hypophyseal trophic hormones. Only secretion of ACTH requires intervention of the hypothalamus *(barred arrow)*.

I. — AGENESIS

Agenesis of the pituitary, that is, absence of the anterior and neural lobes, is seen in human or experimental cyclocephalus. It is apparently due to initial disturbance of notochordal induction.

Partial agenesis, with presence only of the neural lobe, is rarely seen clinically. It is accompanied by adrenal cortical hypoplasia resulting from disruption of the hypothalamic-anterior pituitary connection (see p. 136).

II. — DOUBLING

Experimental. — In amphibians, birds, and even in mammals, doubling of the pituitary has been produced by riboflavin deficiency, hypervitaminosis A, or some tranquilizers. In such cases, there are two neural lobes and two anterior lobes. Opposite the pituitary is a more or less severe doubling of the anterior end of the notochordal system, thus confirming its role as inductor (fig. 1).

In human pathology, some cases of pituitary doubling have been seen with an otherwise normal cephalic end.

These cases may be considered minor forms of double monsters (conjoined twins).

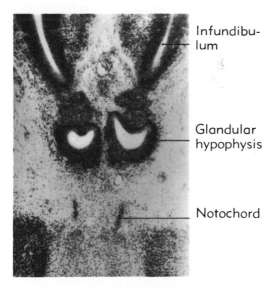

Infundibulum

Glandular hypophysis

Notochord

Fig. 1. — *Hypophyseal doubling in the rat* (according to GIROUD).

MALFORMATIONS

III. — CRANIOPHARYNGIOMAS

Craniopharyngiomas are tumors which especially affect children. They usually develop anterior to the anterior lobe of the pituitary, resulting in visual problems through compression of the optic chiasma. They may be caused by development of the juxtaglandular portion of the pituitary stalk which has failed to regress. The structure of these tumors is generally heterogeneous and very different from that of the glandular hypophysis. The unusual development undergone by these tumors is indicated by the presence of varying mesenchymal tissues within a small area. Intra- and perihypophyseal mesenchyme, ectomesenchyme (leptomeninges), and entomesenchyme (pouch of Seessel) may be seen. The craniopharyngiomas are operable.

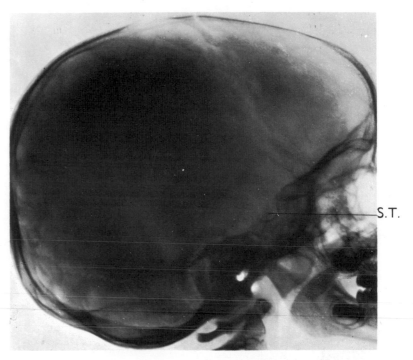

Fig. 2. — *Rœntgenograph of skull profile of a normal 5-year old child.* (S.T. = sella turcica).

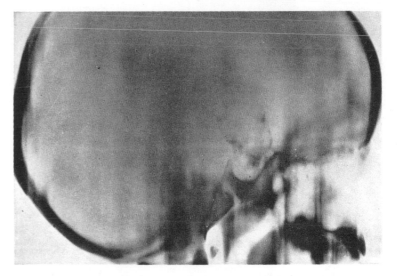

Fig. 3. — *Sagittal tomograph (sectional X-ray) of skull of 4 1/2-year old child with a craniopharyngioma.* The sella turcica is slightly enlarged and intra- and suprasellar calcification of the tumor may be seen. (According to ROUGERIE and FARDEAU.)

THE PARAGANGLIONIC

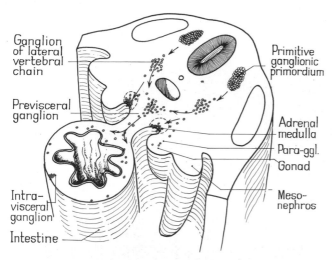

Fig. 1. — *Glandular derivation of the autonomic nervous system* : adrenal medulla and paraganglia. (According to GIROUD and LELIÈVRE, modified.)

The primordial cells of the sympathetic ganglia, or sympathogonia, are not all transformed into nervous cells. Some migrate beyond the sympathetic chain and take on a glandular character (fig. 1 and 2). They form the paraganglionic system, so called because the paraganglia are frequently associated with the sympathetic ganglia and their cells are also derived from the sympathogonia. The mechanism of regulation of this migration is still unknown.

Paraganglionic tissue is found dispersed, in the paraganglia themselves, and in a localized form, the adrenal medulla.

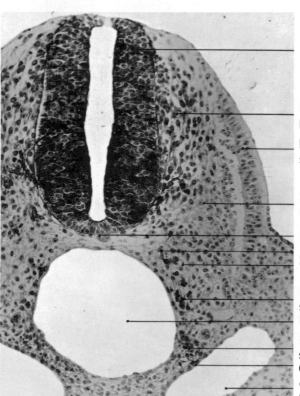

Neural tube

Primitive ganglionic primordium

External portion of somite

Sclerotome cells in migration

Notochord

Sympathogonia

Primordium of sympathetic ganglion
Dorsal aorta

Paraganglionic sympathogonia
Germinative coelomic epithelium
Coelom

Fig. 2. — *Migration of sympathogonia in a 12-day rat embryo* (× 180). (Stained for alkaline phosphatase.)

SYSTEM

THE PARAGANGLIA

During the 2nd month, the sympathogonia detach themselves from the sympathetic primordium and differentiate into glandular cells. Small groups of cells are thus formed behind the peritoneum, in the connective tissue capsule of the adrenal, in the thoracic and abdominal sympathetic chains, in the genital glands, in the epicardium, and elsewhere.

Many of these paraganglia regress when the adrenal medulla becomes functional after birth (for example, the preaortic ganglion of Zuckerkandl situated at the point of emergence of the inferior mesenteric artery). However, large cell clusters persist. They are fragmented, and the resulting paraganglia come in contact with sympathetic ganglionic cells or some blood vessels.

Role of the paraganglia. — The major function of the paraganglia is production of adrenalin or noradrenalin. In the fetus, these two hormones are secreted towards the end of the 4th month. They maintain fetal blood pressure at an optimal level. After birth, this function is taken over by the adrenal medulla and the autonomic nervous system.

Some paraganglia are found near the vagus. They secrete acetylcholine. Their cells do not show the same staining reaction as those of the adrenalin-producing paraganglia, which selectively take up chromium salts (chromaffin reaction).

Paraganglionic tissue liberates adrenalin and acetylcholine more abundantly than do ordinary nerve endings. This specialized tissue may be considered to be in support of organs which function continuously like the heart, or in the vasosensory reflex system which controls circulation.

Pathology: pheochromocytoma or paraganglioma. — Paraganglioma is a tumor involving the paraganglionic system. It may affect the adrenal medulla or the adrenalin-producing paraganglia. There is sometimes abnormal persistence of the organ of Zuckerkandl, which becomes tumorous. The most frequent symptomatology is paroxysmal hypertension.

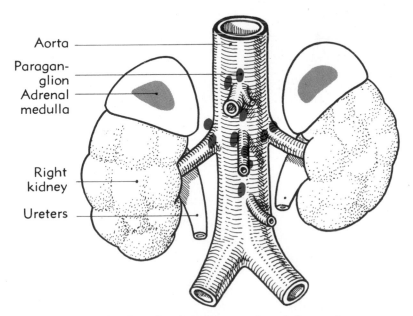

Aorta
Paraganglion
Adrenal medulla
Right kidney
Ureters

Fig. 3. — *Paraganglionic tissue of the renal area in a 6-month old fetus.* (According to PATTEN.)

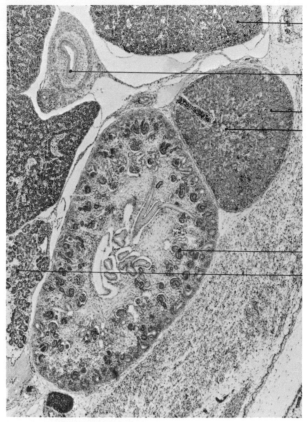

Liver

Intestine

Cortex ⎫
Medulla ⎬

Kidney

Pancreas

Fig. 1. — *Sagittal section of renal area in an 18-day rat fetus* (× 40).

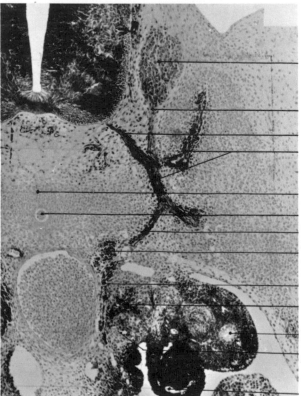

Spinal ganglion

Sensory root

Motor root
Mixed nerve
Vertebral primordium
Notochord
Sympathetic network
Sympathetic ganglion
Sympathogonia and sympathetic nerve networks
Medullary primordium
Renal primordium
Cortical primordium
Gonadal primordium

ADRENAL

ADRENAL

The adrenals are glandular masses found above the kidneys and formed of a cortical zone of mesodermal origin and a medullary zone of ectodermal origin.

The cortical primordium comes from a wide plate of coelomic epithelium in the most internal area of the mesonephric blastema, between the mesenteric root and the gonadal primordium (fig. 2 and 3, and fig. 2, p. 130) [1]. At the beginning of the 2nd month (8 mm), apparently under induction by the primary ureter (Wolffian duct), cell cords form from the epithelium, then penetrate the subjacent mesenchyme.

The medullary primordium results from the assembling of sympathogonia from the sympathetic chain at the mesodermal primordium (fig. 2 and fig. 1, p. 130). This occurs about the 45th day.

[1] This origin explains the existence of accessory paratesticular or paraovarian adrenal cortical masses. In this connection, note that the cortical primordium, cells of the mesonephros, and cells of the gonadal medulla are apparently all derived from the mesonephric blastema.

Fig. 2. — *Cross section of the adrenal area in a 15-day rat fetus* (× 85).

DEVELOPMENT

Adrenal primordium. — About the 50th day (embryo about 20 mm), the two primordia intertwine and the sympathogonia invade the mesodermal primordium. Next, perhaps under the influence of this invasion, the meso- dermal cells multiply quickly and completely surround the medullary pri- mordium. They form the fetal cortex, so called because it regresses after birth ([1]).

Before the 5th month the cortex seems to develop rather autonomously. After this time, its development depends on hypophyseal coricotrophic hormone (ACTH).

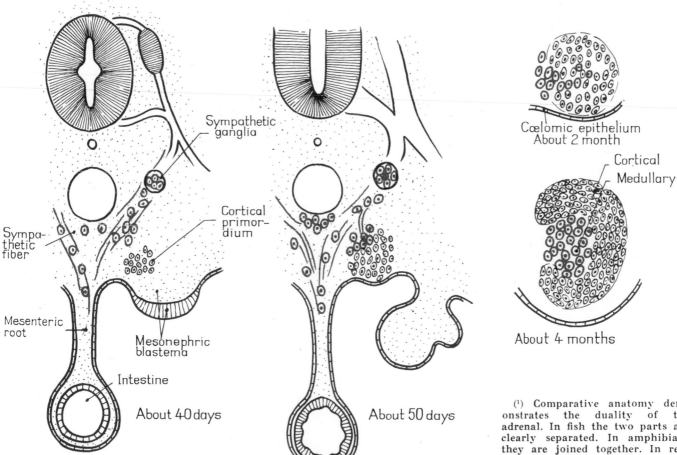

Fig. 3. — *Development of the adrenal in man.*
(According to HAMILTON, BOYD, and MOSSMAN.)

([1]) Comparative anatomy dem- onstrates the duality of the adrenal. In fish the two parts are clearly separated. In amphibians they are joined together. In rep- tiles and birds they tend to fuse unsystematically. Only mammals have the cortical-medullary struc- ture.

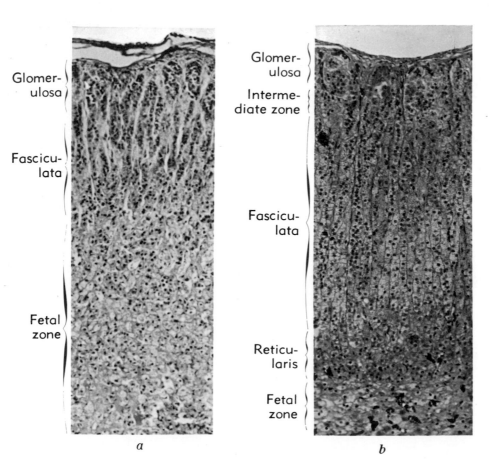

Connective tissue capsule

D.C.

F.Z.

D.C.

Central Medulla vein

Fig. 1. — Section of adrenal of a newborn.
D.C. : primordium of definitive cortex; F.Z. : fetal zone.

After the fetal cortex is formed, the coelomic epithelium gives rise to a second cellular proliferation towards the end of the 3rd month. Small basophilic cells rapidly cover the fetal cortex, whose cells are large and acidophilic. They form the primordium of the definitive cortex, where the future glomerular and fascicular zones are soon differentiated (fig. 1 and 2 *a*). This first differentiation seems to be independent of any hypophyseal stimulation. The reticular zone appears only after birth.

In a parallel way, the medullary cells assemble in the center of the gland (fig. 1).

At birth, the medulla is only slightly developed and not yet functional. The definitive cortex is only a peripheral ring representing 15 to 20% of the glandular parenchyma. The structure of the external glomerular zone is still imprecise, but the zona fasciculata is easily recognizable. It is directly continuous with the fetal zone (fig. 2 *a*).

Glomer-
ulosa

Fascicu-
lata

Fetal
zone

a

Glomer-
ulosa

Interme-
diate zone

Fascicu-
lata

Reticu-
laris

Fetal
zone

b

Fig. 2. — Section of human adrenal.

a) In a newborn (higher magnification of figure 1).

b) Two and one-half months after birth.

THE ADRENAL

The fetal zone begins to regress (pyknosis and lipid degeneration), but does not disappear completely until the second year (fig. 3).

While this regression is taking place, the zonae glomerulosa and fasciculata develop and the reticularis appears (fig. 2 b). It is currently thought that the intermediate zone, between the glomerulosa and fasciculata, is the origin of the 3 types of cortical cells. Development of the definitive cortex and its physiological activity seems to be largely regulated by ACTH.

The adrenal cortex is not completely differentiated until 18 to 24 months after birth (fig. 3).

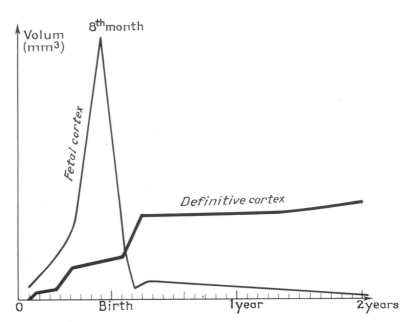

Fig. 3. — Pre- and postnatal development of the adrenal cortex.

Vascularization

The adrenal arteries come from the abdominal aortic system. Upon reaching the gland, they ramify and some reach the medulla directly. The majority nourish the extended capillary network of the glomerulosa and reticularis. The blood then flows into the vessels of the medulla, and leaves it by a large central vein (fig. 1), which emerges at the hilus of the gland. There are thus important vascular relationships between cortex and medulla. (Some compounds of cortical origin, such as vitamin C and cortisone, seem to be necessary for the synthesis of adrenalin).

Innervation

Preganglionic sympathetic ramifications (they do not make synapses in a sympathetic ganglion) reach the center of the coelomic cortical primordium with the sympathogonia (fig. 4). This organization allows assimilation of the adrenal medulla and the other paraganglia to the postganglionic sympathetic neurons. Many sympathetic ganglion cells are found in the medulla.

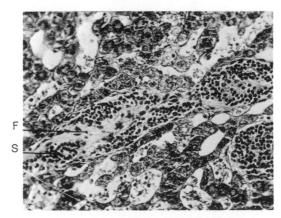

Fig. 4. — Sympathetic nervous fibers (F) and sympathogonia (S) in the cortical primordium. Human fetus of about 2 1/2 months.

I. — PHYSIOLOGY

Development of the adrenal reveals:

1. **The sympathetic nature of the medullary cells.** — This origin explains their production of adrenalin.

2. **The close contact of these cells with the sympathetic nervous system.** — This neuroendocrine device permits extremely rapid reactions, like discharges of adrenalin during stress.

3. **The relationship between the cortical coelomic primordium and the sex gland.** — This relationship explains the production by the fetal and adult cortex of hormones of similar or even indentical composition to those of the gonads.

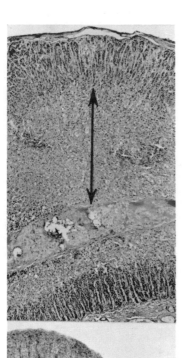

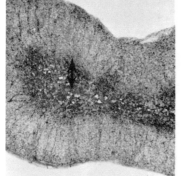

The physiological role of the fetal zone is not currently established. It is known that it produces steroid hormones (androgens in particular) and cortical hormones in small quantities (hydrocortisone), but the purpose of this production is not known.

The functions of the definitive cortex are much better known. The glomerulosa produces mineral corticoids (aldosterone), and under the stimulation of ACTH, the fasciculata produces glucocorticoids (hydrocortisone). The reticularis furnishes sex hormones.

II. — PATHOLOGY

1. The pituitary-adrenal combination in the anencephalic

In anencephalics the anterior pituitary is often only slightly affected, but since the hypothalamus is destroyed, the neurohypophysis does not contain neurosecretion. Without this, ACTH is not secreted, even in the presence of an intact anterior lobe (fig. 2). This situation has little effect before the 5th month, since development of the adrenal seems to be autonomous. After this time, however, development of the fetal cortex cannot take place without ACTH. In the anencephalic there is therefore an involution of the cortex (fig. 1, *arrows*).

The future definitive cortex shows only a simple retardation of development (fig. 1, D.C.), for it is relatively independent of ACTH in the fetus.

NOTE: In the hydrocephalic, the hypothalamus is undamaged, and the adrenals are normally developed.

Fig. 1. — *Adrenal of normal newborn (above) and of anencephalic (below).* D.C. : primordium of definitive cortex.

OF THE ADRENAL

Fig. 2. — *Neuroendocrine correlations in an anencephalic.* Only the fetal cortex is affected. The other glands show only a small retardation of development. (According to Lacomme, Tuchmann-Duplessis and Mercier-Parot.)

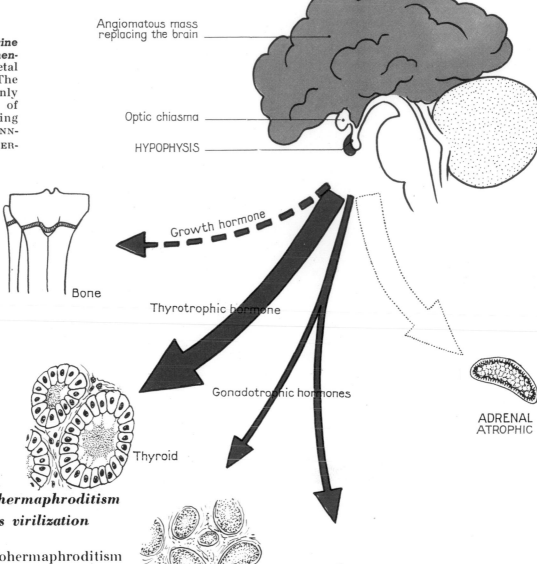

2. *Female pseudohermaphroditism and precocious virilization*

Female pseudohermaphroditism produces late fetal masculanization of the female genital tract. Ovary, uterus, and Fallopian tubes are present, but the vagina opens into a sinus which has developed into a ureter, and a prostate is also present. The hypertrophied clitoris forms a small penis whose groove has remained open (hypospadias). Derivatives of the Wolffian duct are not found.

This masculinization is due to an abnormally high secretion of androgens by the fetal zone or the definitive cortex (urine analyses at birth). The fetal zone may be tumorous, but usually it is the cortex which is hypertrophied. This is the situation in the Debré-Fibiger syndrome where there is hyperplasia of the fascicular and reticular layers.

This rather frequent anomaly is of genetic origin. Transmission is autosomal recessive and the genotype of the subject is actually female (XX).

In the male hypermasculinization produces precocious virilization.

INDEX (*)

(*) Heavy type indicates main sections.

MASSON et Cie, Editeurs,
120, Bd St-Germain, Paris (VIe).
Dépôt légal 2e trimestre 1975

Printed in France

Composition
UNION TYPOGRAPHIQUE
94 Villeneuve St Georges
Achevé d'imprimé sur les Presses
de l'Imprimerie Fécomme
11, 13 ruelle des Champs
77 Villeparisis
Dépôt légal 2e trimestre 1975
N° 1002